The Practice of Mental Health Nursing:

A Community Approach

The Practice of Mental Health Nursing:
A Community Approach

Arthur James Morgan, M.D.
Director of Adult Services
Pennsylvania Hospital
Community Mental Health Center
Philadelphia

Judith Wilson Moreno, R.N., M.S.N.
Director of Out-Patient Department
Pennsylvania Hospital
Community Mental Health Center
Philadelphia

J. B. LIPPINCOTT COMPANY
Philadelphia • Toronto

Distributed in Great Britain by
Blackwell Scientific Publications
London • Oxford • Edinburgh

Paperbound: ISBN-0-397-54148-1
Clothbound: ISBN-0-397-54142-2

Library of Congress Catalog Card Number   73-1622

Printed in the United States of America

4 6 8 9 7 5 3

Library of Congress Cataloging in Publication Data

Morgan, Arthur James
    The practice of mental health nursing.

    Includes bibliographies.
    1. Psychiatric nursing. 2. Community mental health services. I. Moreno, Judith Wilson, joint author. II. Title. [DNLM: 1. Community mental health services. 2. Psychiatric nursing. WY 160 M847p 1973]

RC440.M67   610.73'68   73-1622
ISBN 0-397-54142-2
ISBN 0-397-54148-1 (P)

To Mary

—A.J.M.

To Susan, Jamie, Molly and Vete for their
patience, support and good humor

—J.W.M.

CONTENTS

Acknowledgments

The authors are grateful to the Pennsylvania Hospital and its Community Mental Health Center for their wisdom in giving the staff the professional freedom to develop their own techniques and methods to deal with the special challenges of this new delivery system of mental health services.

We wish to thank Roger B. Daniels, M.D., Department of Medicine, Pennsylvania Hospital, for his help in reviewing the medical accuracy of Chapter 10.

We are also grateful to the J. B. Lippincott Company for its vision and courage in supporting this innovative approach, especially David T. Miller, Vice President, J. B. Lippincott Company, who in his delightful way would press us to rework sections time and again by saying, "That's very good, but I still don't know how to do a psychiatric interview (or crisis intervention)." We relied on his experience and were encouraged by his faith in the project.

Finally we thank Mary Dennesaites, Editor, Nursing Department, J. B. Lippincott Company, who "saw" the book long before we had written it and encouraged and assisted us for untold hours to "say it like it is," to write from our experiences, and to write it in English. Her sensitivity and compassion in handling the material we presented was also extended towards the reader, and beyond that, to the patients we are all struggling to help.

A.J.M.
J.W.M.

Introduction

THE PRACTICE OF MENTAL HEALTH NURSING: A COMMUNITY APPROACH marks a revolutionary departure from traditional nursing, psychiatric and medical textbooks of the past. Not bound to any one school of thought or theoretical frame of reference, our orientation is derived from actual clinical practice and experience in the community mental health movement since its inception. An attempt has been made to present all necessary information in a clear and lively fashion including the basic facts which are often so tedious and boring to learn. Those things the student unfortunately must memorize are labeled "things you unfortunately must memorize. Memorize them."

The authors feel the presentation of factual information in palatable form is but a small part of their task. What we have attempted to do is to think and to interact with the student, to anticipate questions and hesitations, to encourage original thought, and to encourage the student to press ahead where it is safe to do so.

As we wrote the book we clearly remembered our student days in psychiatry, the one in a psychiatric residency and the other in a M.S.N. program, and reminded ourselves that we never had a book like this but that this was exactly what we had wanted. No one would ever say how therapy was done or what mental illness was all about in terms that related to our life experiences at the time. Everything was a little mystical and scary and we had to put off our understanding of what was really going on until much later in our professional careers.

What we learned is in this book. What we found out, of course, is that mental health or psychiatric work is exactly like anything else in the world. There is no magic to be learned, no state of exalted awareness or pure health for the therapist and no necessary snake pit of despair for the patient.

The first step in our personal growth towards our present understanding* was in giving ourselves the right to drop the professional jargon, the mumbo jumbo that mystifies, intimidates and confuses.

The next was to think of and relate to our patients as people. Patients often insist, despite profound professional pressure, on being people with unique problems. If somebody you know is doing some-

---

*This evolution for both of us occurred separately and before we began working together at the same center.

thing stupid, you say "Hey, that's stupid, stop it." Our training directed us not to think of or speak to our patients like this, for reasons that were never too clear. It had something to do with imposing our value system on the patient or directing him, instead of allowing him the dignity of discovering his own path.

Well, sooner or later, especially in the clear reality of a community mental health center we dropped the passive pose and blurted out a "Hey, that's stupid, stop it." The patient stopped.

Gradually we learned to differentiate between those people who want and need direction and straight talk and those who need gentler handling. Instead of a flute and an oboe we assembled a whole orchestra of instruments to interpret the score of life, no matter how it is written.

One overwhelming advantage to working in a community mental health center is the rich professional mix and variety of training and experience that the workers bring to their job. It is, albeit irritating and frustrating at first, in the long run both refreshing and stimulating to the Freudian to hear one case discussed in Sullivanian terms, another in Jungian, to have a young psychiatrist insist on the terms of transactional analysis, to have a social worker be on a strictly Maslow trip, and then have a mental health worker propose that both staff and patients practice meditation (following which proposal, twenty of the staff begin meditating to see for themselves).

This ferment of opinion and controversy brings up concepts and possibilities that never would come to mind in an ordinary setting with a particular orientation.

The community mental health center, in spite of its total and comprehensive approach, is not in any sense the total Institution described by Groff in *Asylums*. It is, in fact, the antithesis of this. The patients continue living in and dealing with the real world in which they got sick. They come in with some very practical problems and some very real needs that do not lend themselves to theoretical discussion or esoteric elaboration of the point of view held by a school of thought. Practical problems like poverty, malnutrition, and rats and filth in the house require practical, immediate solutions like money, food, and the services of an exterminator, as well as the department of Licenses and Inspections. There is no place for theoretical constructs or encouraging the patient to "work it out for himself" in these situations. Terms like "hostile environment" and "quality of life" take on an entirely new meaning in a poverty situation. Words like "crisis" and "emergency" also come alive in a very special way.

The result of this interdisciplinary mix of staff, with a loud and clear input from patients and community who know what "trouble" is, is a very practical, down-to-earth approach.

The philosophy that emerges is existentialism. The therapy is reality-oriented. The emphasis is on life-in-the-world, the quality of it and the joy of it.

The patient is central in the community mental health center and in this book. The "patient" is frequently an entire family, or a married couple, or a parent and child and occasionally a separate individual.

We have emphasized the role of the center in the delivery of mental health services, that is to say, in direct patient care. That is our area of competence and expertise as therapists, educators, and administrators, and we feel that almost all other workers in the community mental health system are also oriented this way. Other areas of a center's function (by federal mandate) are Research and Evaluation and Consultation and Education. There are few centers in the country today with viable, fully operating, effective departments of Research and Evaluation and Consultation and Education, and it is unlikely that the nurse would have much contact with them. Research and Evaluation is usually done by trained researchers—research psychologists, statisticians, and biometricians. It would be most helpful to get some really good studies under way that would tell us in five or ten years how we are doing, how effective we really are, and where we might modify our programs to become more effective. Unfortunately, these studies are just beginning. Consultation and Education is involved in primary prevention: It is intended to increase good mental health practices in the community through schools and other institutions so that the actual incidence (number of new cases per year per unit population) of mental illness will drop. In our experience, Consultation and Education departments seldom flourish because they immediately run into two blocks that we do not have the skills to tackle as yet. One is poverty, the other is the genetic basis for mental disease. There is also a question, variously answered, as to what extent the government-funded center can get into an all-out war with other government-funded agencies like Housing and Urban Development and the Department of Welfare.

Even if such confrontations are entered in the name of patients' rights, there is a serious question about what can be accomplished at that level. A larger social plan is necessary to make a real dent in the incidence of mental disorder, and society is not yet ready to appreciate or take this step.

Of the delivery modalities within the community mental health system two have enjoyed an outstanding growth and appear to have permanently changed the face of psychiatric practice. They are crisis intervention and the partial hospital. The authors have been directly involved in the development of these two services and write from experience and with considerable conviction. Psychiatry in the office and psychiatry in the hospital are both diminishing rapidly. Intervention in the home, on the street, or wherever necessary, and alternatives to hospitalization are the tools of today. This "new psychiatry" is not at all confined to the mental health center. Almost all private and public mental hospitals have begun a partial hospitalization service and many are starting crisis intervention. The emphasis on these services should be most valuable to the student and the nurse regardless of the setting in which clinical experience is obtained.

The actual de-emphasis of the specifics of inpatient care may lead some students to feel they will not therefore be prepared to work on an inpatient ward. This is not true. Former specifics of inpatient care such as techniques and indications for physical restraints and postinsulin or psychosurgery are rarely required to be known today. Seclusion room care and various degrees of suicide precaution are used occasionally, vary from hospital to hospital, and can be learned in a few minutes of ward instruction. Other than these, there is little difference between the milieu and therapeutic thrust made on an inpatient ward and that made in a partial hospital setting.

The popular phrase "team approach" is mentioned only in passing in this book, and is rather conspicuous by its absence in a textbook on community mental health. This is because all of the "teams" that the authors have seen have emphasized careful role definition and have tended toward something of an assembly line approach with the patient (or family) moving down a conveyer belt while the doctor performed one function, the nurse the other, the social worker another and so forth. We find this to be an artificial subdivision of labor and responsibility and not a natural arrangement at all. We find that while it is true that one person can do something better than another, this difference has much less to do with training and "professional role" than with the individual's own capabilities, personality, and interests. One nurse may have a particular flair for psychopharmacology and another may detest it; one really takes to home visiting and crisis intervention and another finds these things tedious. The same personality differences, of course, hold true for psychiatrists, social workers, mental health workers, psychiatric technicians, and others.

As we wrote we tried starting sentences such as "The nurse's role in crisis intervention is . . ." or ". . . in the intake process is . . ." and we gave up, deleting this structure altogether. It just is not the way things work in reality. We have visited centers where careful role definition is valued highly and found almost everyone doing things that he or she did not do well and did not want to do, with the net result that the productivity of the center was very low and the mood of the center was one of "fulfilling a professional responsibility" rather than one of cheerful enthusiasm.

So, if you read this book to try to determine the "nurse's role" in community mental health, you will not find it here. Instead you will find a steady insistence on a *colleague relationship* between the nurse and doctor. When the nurse is better at diagnosis or administration or group therapy than the doctor, then these are the things she does. Because they work closely together, the doctor and nurse both know what the other's interests and capabilities are: they trust one another in their area of competence and question one another in areas of less competence; they learn from one another; they respect each other.

There are of course a few legally determined functions that doctors must perform (like prescription writing) and things that nurses must do (like giving injections), but these occupy less than ten percent of the day. These duties are simply accepted as necessary and unavoidable and we try to do them quickly and well. Even these, however, are usually done *together,* with the doctor and nurse collaborating on medication decisions and both talking a patient into a necessary injection and both giving it. We feel this arrangement is healthy and right. It is, after all, what we tell our patients to do when we say "find out what you like to do and what you are good at—and do that. Get in touch with your feelings and go with them."

In this book the nurse will also find many advanced concepts of clinical practice discussed that are usually reserved for study in graduate programs. This is deliberate. We believe that "advanced concepts" tend to include all the "good stuff" and exciting material while "basic concepts" generally are confined to the dullest, most boring aspects of the subject. The trend in education is toward the approach we have taken. It turns out to be possible to learn the alphabet and spelling and grammar *while* reading an interesting story, instead of memorizing all the dull stuff first. As a matter of fact, it turns out to be a better, more effective teaching method to be exposed to the whole Gestalt from the very beginning. Adequate warnings are given so that the student does not plunge in over her head prematurely. We trust the student's judgment to heed these.

1
Professional Jargon

Psychiatry is rich in jargon which must be learned if one is to move into the world of the knowing ones and speak the language that is spoken there. However, words which are invented to express concepts and theoretical constructs and to clarify communication quickly become the password to professional acceptance and take on meanings that their inventors never intended. Before long they cloud communication and serve a counterproductive (note the jargon) purpose.

Freud, for example, found it convenient to think of the functions of the mind as being in three general categories. The *ego* functions (the "I") embrace those which we generally think of as being "ourselves." The *id* functions (the "it") consist of the animal instincts within us such as our drives, lusts and so forth. The *super-ego* (the "other I") is a category of mental functioning that has to do with conscience, control, and certain prohibitions. Freud envisioned the id as being powerful, gross and totally unreasonable, striving to keep its owner alive, fed, and sexually gratified whatever the cost. The super-ego would tend to oppose these crude, selfish impulses of the id and, like the voice of the parents, (only inside the self) says such things as "That's not nice," "Say you're sorry," "Don't get dirty," "Don't hurt your sister," and "Don't touch yourself there." The ego is the function that takes the real world into account (what can and can't be done) and tries to resolve the conflict that the id and super-ego functions are always having. If the id desires you to pick up a large rock and kill someone who is in your way and the super-ego is shouting "murderer," "selfish beast," "monster," the ego may consider something more realistic like walking around the person while observing that the rock is probably too heavy to lift and that it doesn't make sense to strain yourself and take a chance of going to jail or getting yourself killed by the other guy anyway. The ego is a mediator, is social, is reasonable. The id is none of these. The super-ego is social only, but in a very rigid and unreasonable way. We are born with an id, develop an ego and acquire a super-ego.

All well and good. Viewing the mind in this way has been of very great help in understanding personality development and how distortions occur. It is probably the most widely accepted scheme around.

However, these words (id, ego, super-ego) have become household words for many and are misused by professionals and nonprofessionals alike. "Bill's on an ego trip" means something like self-aggrandizement, having too much pride, having a ball over how great you are. "She can use some ego" means she has a feeling of low self-esteem. "He has too rigid a super-ego" means he is too hard on himself. "Honey, I can't keep the lid on my id around you" means "Let's have sex." The words are used far differently than Freud intended. They now imply components of a personality or certain kinds of mental behavior rather than functions of the mind. They have become part of the vocabulary of idle conversation and are of very little use to us today in really understanding what is going on with a person.

To make matters worse, community psychiatry and nursing have adopted much of the jargon of public health, sociology, psychology, theology, philosophy and the Federal Bureaucracy. In staff meetings of some centers, English is hardly spoken at all.

In our work and in this book, we have tried as far as possible to return to the English language. It is after all what most of our patients speak, and it is what we ourselves use at home and with our friends. It has been difficult, and we have not been totally successful. In our work we have been helped by our patients who hold to the not unreasonable idea that they not only want to know what we are saying and feeling but that they have the right to know. We agree. With professional colleagues such help is not as readily available. Upon hearing English spoken, some professionals cry "superficial," "lacking in depth," "undignified," "unscientific." These professionals, however, are people too. To help the student in dealing with them we present their language—not all of it, but enough to give some vocabulary and phrases to "get by" in their country.

Where possible we will give both the original usage and the popular usage (as in the "ego" example) so that the nurse will understand both "dialects." Use it as we suggest, use it for examination purposes, but for heaven's sake, don't start to think about yourselves, your friends or the people we call patients in this language.

Client: A person who is buying professional services such as legal services or interior design services. Used as a substitute for "patient" by some mental health professionals who oppose the "medical model" of mental disorder.

Guest: Used as another euphemism for "patient," especially in homes for the elderly.

Medical Model: A phrase of derision used by psychologists, social workers and others when referring to the way nurses and doctors approach patients. It implies that medically trained personnel do not consider patients as people but as subjects who have acquired a disease process, and who need medical attention. It implies that the social aspects and behavioral aspects of a patient are not taken into consideration. Generally those who oppose "medical model" prefer "psychological model" or "educational model" and similarly would substitute "client" for "patient" and "education" for "treatment." (This absurd quarrel is quickly ended by speaking English.)

Etiology: Cause or causative elements for something.

Dynamics: An explanation of the forces (usually unconscious) that are presumed to be at work in a patient which result in the particular symptoms or manifestations that are seen. The question is asked in this way: "Miss Smith, would you please discuss the dynamics of this patient's paranoid productions with special attention to the developmental history and etiologic factors as you understand them?" Translation: "Do you know a theory about what causes someone to become suspicious and feel persecuted, and does this patient seem to fit the theory?" The student quickly learns that use of the word "dynamics" often indicates that the instructor has a notion about what causes a certain set of symptoms, and that it would be helpful for academic well-being to determine what the instructor's frame of reference is regarding "dynamics."

Theory, belief and truth: These three valuable words are included here not because they constitute jargon but because their value is so often diminished by misuse. There are no truths in psychiatry, community or otherwise. Truth here means that what we say and think about the mind of man is an accurate reflection of what the mind really is. What we have, and what allows us to act at all, are ideas, theories, and/or concepts of the mind which make some sense to us. When our actions, based on theory, bring the results we anticipate and want, we tend to believe that the theory has some aspect of truth in it. There are psychoanalytic, behavioral and biochemical theories of the mind on which very different therapeutic approaches are based, and all have some measure of success; thus, all may contain some aspect of truth. The proponents of these theories often *believe* them and behave as though they were *truth*.

Eclectic: Means "freely choosing." Properly refers to the therapist who does not exclusively follow a particular theory of the mind or school of thought but chooses elements from a number of theories that are pleasing to, and work for, the therapist. Its misuse comes when it serves to cover ignorance as to the theoretical basis of therapeutic action. If you have your own theoretical scheme which guides your therapeutic efforts, do not call it "eclectic." Call it your own and define it for yourself and others.

Learning: An excellent word from the field of education that, like the term "ego" from psychiatry, has been so abused that it no longer conveys anything useful. There is learning theory, student-centered learning, teacher-centered learning; there are learning methods, learning labs, learning workshops, learning techniques, *ad infinitum*.

Process: An organized, consistent, interrelated series of steps from one level of development or organization to another, as in the healing process or the growth process. A favorite word of some who say "Today we will discuss process in therapy" and group dynamics people who speak about "group process." These mean, respectively, the steps that the patient and therapist must take in therapy when following a particular theory, and the steps by which a collection of people become a group and establish group goals, standards, feelings, etc.

On-going: Means simply "continuing," as opposed to "limited." "Is she in on-going therapy?" means "Is her therapy continuing?" A classical example of mental health jargon.

Normal: Means something like "common" or "expected" or "ordinary." Being the opposite of "abnormal" has probably hurt the word more than anything and given it a strong moralistic and judgmental flavor. "Uncommon," "unexpected," and "extraordinary" do not hurt their opposites in this negative way. "Normal" should probably never be used because it is too damaging.

Projection: A perfectly fine word used by Freud to describe one of the mechanisms by which the ego protects itself by ascribing one's own unconscious motivations to another. Used as a swear word by many professionals when speaking with each other. "I think Sue is afraid of men" (this is my valid impression). "You're projecting" (you are the one who is afraid of men but you don't know it and you blame Sue instead. Your impression and your thinking on the subject are entirely invalid). When "You're projecting" is delivered with a knowing, even "understanding" smile, it's time to walk away. Banter of this sort is probably initiated by insecure people (as is most banter) but because the game is destructive it should not be played.

Neurotic: A pejorative word in such common usage as to make its professional use (it still has one) quite difficult. "I don't want to go skydiving." "You're neurotic." Used in this example, it means timid, stupid, fretful, different from others (odd), like others (conforming) and many other things. It should not be generally used. Professionally it refers to syndromes which constitute minor mental illness as compared to major mental illness (psychotic, or the psychoses). For those who think of the psychoses as organic, the neuroses are functional (psychologically caused). It should be noted that some neuroses are more incapacitating than some psychoses, just as some infections are more incapacitating than some cancers.

Paranoid: Overused and misused. Another professional swear word. Rightly refers to a specific symptom complex where the patient loses the distinction between what is happening in himself and what is happening in the world, and perceives danger where there is none. "I'm not paranoid, I'm really persecuted" is as good a retort as any to its pejorative use.

Functional: Okay to use when the intention is to ascribe to a syndrome psychological causes as opposed to organic (physical) causes. Be sure to recognize that this distinction is only theoretical and may have to be abandoned altogether in the future.

Rationalization: Another swear word. In proper usage it is applied to a patient's attempt to explain in reasonable terms his behavior or thoughts which happened unreasonably (unconsciously). We all use this mechanism and rightly resent having it pointed out to us as a put-down. Nor should we use it in this way. The girl in group therapy who says she would rather read than date boys may indeed rather read. If she has a free choice between the two (i.e., both are available) then her "rather read" is not a rationalization even though we ourselves might make a different choice.

Authority problem: (As in "Joe has an authority problem.") The misuse of this phrase consists of its being applied to anyone who can't get along with or who dislikes someone in authority. Properly used it describes a person who chronically and continuously has trouble with those in authority, benign though they may be. The ability to distinguish between good, capable bosses and weak, ineffective bosses and to perceive a boss's personality characteristics is worthy of developing and is a sound attribute. It does not in any way imply an "authority problem." Could it be that people who always talk of others' authority problems are projecting?

Counterdependent: Means an attitude of a basically dependent person which is developed to hide his dependency from himself and others and involves being antagonistic to any offers to help or lead or direct or teach him. The term is just beginning to be misused in the field.

I.P.: From family therapy theory. Means the "Identified Patient," or the family member who represents the family and displays its pathology. Is used as jargon: "Beginning with the I.P., the undifferentiated ego mass of the R. family was gradually delineated."

Therapeutic Self: This term appears to represent that portion of a psychiatric nurse which is used to help a patient, e.g.: "primarily utilizing my therapeutic self a successful intervention was accomplished, considerably lessening the patient's suicide potential." Translation: "I talked to the guy like a human being and he felt better" or "I let the patient know I really cared and it helped a lot."

The reader is referred to the Glossary for formal definitions of commonly used psychiatric words and phrases.

2

The Psychiatric Interview

The first step in learning the skills of interviewing is to gain some understanding of the patient's feelings when he decides to seek professional help. Consider the following description of a not uncommon situation and think about each event, how you might respond, and how you would feel.

You have always been a fairly good student, but you have noticed an increasing tendency to daydream during lectures and when you try to study it is difficult to concentrate. Your grades are falling. Although you are concerned, you try not to think about it. Your appetite is less and you've lost weight. At night you watch the late show, though it bores you, because you have difficulty falling asleep. Your interest in things, even your own grooming, has diminished. Your attitude of "Oh! what the hell's the use!" surprises you at times. Your friends begin to ask "What's wrong?" You don't answer, because you aren't sure. You consider dropping out of college, although you are unsure what you would do if you did. You decide to remain in school, but begin to cut almost every class, and you are frightened by what you perceive as a loss of self-control. It seems that anything would be better than the way you feel now. Some of your friends have used LSD and you accept an invitation to a party where you are sure people will be using it. You feel a little exhilarated in anticipation for the first time in a couple of months, and you are scared. You try not to think about it. Your roommate, learning of your party plans, decides to talk to you and does. She enumerates all the changes in your behavior that alarm her and you know she's right. She suggests "Something's wrong" and you agree. Her concern and willingness to "intrude," despite your attempts to prevent her, impress you. She suggests an appointment with a psychiatrist "to talk things over" and indicates you could see one privately (the college has several private consultants) or arrange an appointment at the community mental health center located several blocks away. You decide to skip the party. You cry. You have a fleeting thought that maybe suicide would be "a good solution" and think about it for awhile, even though the idea scares you. You can't get to sleep. You decide you have to get help. You feel confused, depressed, and worried. You just hope "it isn't too late." In the morning you call the community mental health center for an appointment (you realize private care would be too expensive) and you are given an appointment with a nurse for the next day. You are surprised that you won't be seeing a doctor and worry a bit about that. In the morning you walk over to the center, thinking all the way about skipping the appointment. You wonder, "What will I say? What will *she* say? There's nothing wrong—I need to get myself together—I can't do it! This is silly melodrama!" But, you have arrived at the center. You pass by the entrance and stand across the street for a few minutes and watch to see who goes inside and what they look like. The people look "sane" so you decide they must not be patients. You feel embarrassed and wonder if you're mentally ill, and then abruptly cross over and quickly walk into the building. The doors seem awfully heavy. You announce your name to the receptionist and are aware of a pounding sensation in your chest and you are breathing heavily. You sit in a waiting area and cry. You feel shaky, sad, anxious, and relieved.

BACKGROUND OBSERVATIONS

The decision itself to seek psychiatric consultation produces anxiety in many people. In some cultures the treatment of emotional disorder is delegated to the shaman, witch doctor or priest who exercises mystical powers to treat and cure. In such primitive societies there is fear and apprehension associated with the need for consultation and treatment by the local "shrink." When not engaged in active "treatment" these primitive psychotherapists are responsible for interpreting and explaining natural or unnatural phenomena. Modern day psychiatrists and psychotherapists have "inherited" this role. The reaction of the average American to a psychiatric treatment facility and the therapists he will encounter there, while it is hopeful, curious, and optimistic, is also as skeptical, anxious, and fearful as that of his counterpart in past and present primitive cultures.

It is wise to keep in mind that most people seeking help at a community mental health center will not be the sophisticated, intellectual, interesting, and articulate types described by Thomas Mann, F. Scott Fitzgerald, and more recently by Philip Roth.* For the most part the average person seeking treatment at a community mental health center is reacting to a variety of personal and social pressures with which he is unable to cope. Emotional equilibrium is generally impaired, and anxiety, with its discomfort, becomes the almost universal symptom. The initial psychiatric interview with an attentive, sympathetic, and competent therapist will usually result in a reduction of anxiety, thereby giving the patient the feeling of some relief and laying the groundwork for what is to follow. The first interview is critical, and it is easy to understand how its success can affect the outcome of the therapeutic relationship.** It is interesting, but not surprising, to note that most of what has been written concerning the psychiatric interview deals with the interview as performed by a psychiatrist, and not in a community mental health center. Do not be dismayed! The skill and competence to conduct such an interview are not confined to the psychiatrist although this has been the time-honored belief. Recognition of this does not assure change. Community mental health centers operate through local, state, and federal funding which ebbs and flows with political tides. The centers' pressing need for skilled therapists, in tandem with these uncertain financial resources, has spawned innovation that has successfully demonstrated that sensitivity, perception, empathy and therapeutic competence are neither restricted to the psychiatrist nor guaranteed by his training. Nurses, psychologists and social workers have been enlisted to participate in this new-style delivery of psychotherapy. Therapy in a community mental health center is reality-oriented. It is essential for the nurse-therapist in such a setting to be well-informed about available resources in the community and to utilize these to assist the patient coming to her for help. The presenting symptoms are usually psychiatric, but the etiology of the problem may be social or physical rather than just intrapsychic.

THE INTERVIEW

As indicated above, the initial psychiatric interview is crucial. It is a starting point and a time of mixed feelings for the patient. Try to create in your mind the feeling you have as you come to the community mental health center in need of psychiatric consultation.

You are anxious as you wait for the person to whom you will be telling your problems. Your thoughts run together and con-

---

*Author of the popular novel *Portnoy's Complaint*.

**The pivotal nature of this initial psychiatric interview has been discussed and analyzed by prominent therapists in the past and present, and the student is referred to literature available on this subject, in particular the classic by Sullivan, H. S. *The Psychiatric Interview*, New York, Norton, 1954.

tribute to your feeling of confusion. You try to figure out what has happened to cause your present situation, and you have difficulty sorting out "where it started." Some of the anxiety you feel is related to the fear of not knowing what to do or what will happen next. You wonder whether the decision to seek help was too hasty and wonder what will be revealed to the school officials—how confidential will it be? Will your schooling be interrupted? You don't much care about school, or anything, but you wonder what you'll do and how you'll feel if the shrink says, "You need a rest." As you think of these things, and try to hold on to a single thought until you've considered it, you feel exhausted by the effort. You realize your thinking ability has changed. You know how "messed-up" your "head" is, and again question whether you've "flipped out." It occurs to you that things started going downhill after the bout with infectious mononucleosis last summer, but you quickly reject that as insignificant. You can't recall anyone in your family ever being crazy, but then your parents would have "protected" you from that knowledge even if it were true! All these thoughts are like bees swarming around a hive and concentration is so difficult that again you realize how tired and washed-out you feel.

If you were able to formulate the chief concerns you are feeling as you wait, they would be:

What's happening to me?

What's caused this to happen to me?

What's going to happen to me?

A good way to understand what the patient is feeling is to imagine yourself in a similar situation. It is a useful technique and can help to develop greater sensitivity and awareness of the complex and varied feelings people experience in problem situations. Irrelevant questions or comments, which are the hallmark of an insecure, anxious or insensitive interviewer, can thus be eliminated or at least reduced. Likewise, blanket reassurance which is misleading or erroneous can also be eliminated by using this technique to become more sensitive. Consider, as a nurse, how many times you've told a patient that "this won't hurt" or "everything will be all right" or "it doesn't taste bad," when you really had no way of knowing whether your comments were valid and helpful, or were made in an attempt to reassure yourself and allay your own anxiety. It's wise to keep in mind that just as people react differently to physical pain, so they vary in their response to emotional pain. The nurse who assesses and treats psychiatric patients must be familiar with basic theoretical concepts of psychodynamics, psychopathology and psychotherapy. This knowledge will be enhanced by developing sensitivity to the patient's apprehensions, anxieties and fears.

INTERVIEW TECHNIQUE

The task here is to establish rapport with the patient, to get as complete a picture of his life and how his mind is working as possible, to answer for yourself the kinds of questions that are asked on an interview form such as the Mental Status Examination (see page 187), and to do all these things in a natural and comfortable way.

The patient may have nothing to say or, on the other hand, may produce a diary covering every feeling he could record over the past ten years. The tone of the interview should be friendly, with the interviewer clearly in charge, allowing the patient to speak freely as long as pertinent material is being presented, and only interrupting with questions for clarification or to direct the patient's thinking where necessary.

The room should be private and quiet and the interview should proceed without interruptions.

It begins like this. "Mr. Edwin Jones? Sit here. My name is Mrs. Thomas. I'm a psychiatric nurse and we're going to be talking for a while about you, and what's been troubling you, and see how we can help you." (Pause.) "Okay?" (Pause, then continue with or without response.) "First let me check the information I have. You're 33, unmarried, and live at Tenth and Spruce?" (Look up at patient for affirmation.) "Now, can you tell me in a general way what's been going on with you and particularly what made you decide to come in for help?"

At this point the patient is on his own to tell his story in his own words. The nurse listens attentively and responsively by nodding from time to time, saying "uh-huh" and "I see" or "I understand" to let the patient know that he is doing all right and that he is being heard. For the interviewer to sit tight-lipped and totally passive (as is the style of some in the name of being objective or nondirective) is unfeeling and unnecessary.

The patient doesn't know who you are or what you are thinking or what you want to hear. He knows you are somehow connected with the field of psychiatry and are therefore part of the Establishment. By not giving him any clue as to where your head is at, you reinforce his suspicions about your power, your ability to read minds, and your "straight" value system (e.g., everybody should be perfectly sane, utterly responsible, and work). The fact is that you don't possess any magical power, you can't read minds (that's why you ask questions), and you *are* quite human. All the power you have and need derives from being a gentle, concerned person, interested in understanding the person you are talking to. This need not be said in so many words. The patient will get the idea by your thoughtful listening and careful questioning as the interview proceeds, and he will be greatly relieved thereby.

If the patient is psychotic and rambles on about his delusional system he should be stopped as soon as the depth and breadth of his insanity is apparent to you. The man who tells you that he has a transistor radio in his head that warns him when he is in the presence of the anti-christ can be asked how long he has noticed this and how it makes him feel. You don't need a complete transcription of every "broadcast" he has monitored in the past three years. Far more important is to explore how *nonpsychotic* he is. Where is his mental functioning still intact? What ego-strengths does he have that can be counted on in therapy? Good transition comments are "I think I understand enough about this for right now, Mr. Jones. Tell me how you spend your days? What do you like to do?"

While the patient is describing his perceptions of his problems the nurse will have an opportunity to consider how intelligent he seems and how he handles words and language. Does he use *neologisms,* new words that he has invented like "disconcernity," or does he speak in *"word salad"* like, "Even though the green runs jerking happy cloth breaks glass over mud decay war shoots avocadoes scorpion feet . . ."? The nurse will observe how he gestures and carries himself and moves, how he is dressed and presents himself, how he expresses his feelings (affect), whether affect is appropriate to the things he is saying, what his mood is, and whether he is oriented—that is, knowing who he is, where he is, who you are and what time it is (day, month, year).

If this sort of information is not given spontaneously during the early part of the interview, specific questions will have to be asked toward the end.

CRITICAL AREAS

After the patient has reported as much as he can that is of value to you and has filled in the details you have asked for, it is well to move into direct questioning about three critical areas which few patients spontaneously cover in any but the most cursory fashion. They are his work or school experiences, his drug history and his sex life. This can be done simply and easily, just as any other information is gathered. Inexperienced therapists frequently shy away from these subjects, feeling that it will embarrass the patient or knowing that it will embarrass the interviewer. In truth, almost all patients welcome a full and complete survey of their life, if it is sensitively done, and take such completeness as a sign of competence on the part of the therapist. The experience of most medical-surgical nurses regarding questioning of a patient's bowel and bladder habits is that the more specific the question the more valuable the answer. Patients are more often uncertain about what information is important than they are secretive. The question "Are your bowels and bladder normal?" is confusing, and does not lead the patient into giving a detailed description. It may be better to ask, "How often do you pass your water?" "Do you have any difficulty or pain at any time when doing it?" "How many times do you get out of bed at night to go?" "What color is your urine? Dark like cider? Light yellow?" "Does the stream shut off okay or do you dribble after you're done?" "Do you itch or burn when you urinate?" "Do you get enough warning when you have to go or does the urge come on very suddenly?"—and so forth. These detailed questions let the patient know that you know what you are doing, that you mean business, that you are comfortable with the excretory functions as just another area in a person's life which can yield information about him and add to the assessment that will get him healthy more quickly.

Questioning about work or school, drugs and sex, should proceed as easily and naturally, as completely and professionally, as in the above example. As discussed throughout this book, the examiner's attitude determines the outcome. This should convey interest, professional concern, attention to detail, competence, security and comfort in the role of questioner, a matter-of-fact right to know, and innocence. The critical areas should be covered in the order presented here (unless the patient volunteers information that opens a door to questioning in some other sequence).

The reason for this is that most people will more readily and comfortably answer questions about their work than about the drugs they use, and more easily discuss drugs than sex. By starting in the most neutral area and getting the patient into the mood of honesty and completeness in answering, the therapist can more easily move into more sensitive areas, carried by the patient's expectation of forthrightness.

If the patient wants to talk about sex first because that is what bothers him the most, this is all right, and the information obtained this way can help guide the detailed questioning later.

WORK AND SCHOOL HISTORY

The objective is to get a complete picture of how much schooling the patient has had, how he did, how he felt about it, his plans regarding further school, if any, his plans *before* he got sick, his adjustment to the school situation past and/or present, his relationships with his classmates and teachers, his ability to read, concentrate and remember, the attitude of his friends and family to education.

Regarding work: "Do you work? What do you do? How do you like it? How long have you been doing that job? Are there parts of the job that you don't like? What are they? Do you see much of your boss or supervisor? What kind of a guy is he? How do the other guys get along with him? Do you get along okay with the other guys? Which ones don't you like? How long have you been working there? What did you do before? How long do you think you'll be working there? Are you looking around now? Why not (if job isn't good)? Is the boss satisfied with your work? Are you late or out sick very much? How much? Why? When did that start? Would you say that the job contributed to your getting sick, or is it more that getting sick messes up your ability to do the job?"

Obviously the order of the questions and the areas you get into differ with every patient. The above example gives a sense of the appropriate depth of questioning and clearly indicates the wealth of information about the patient's lifestyle that can be gotten from questions about school and work. A diagnosis can often be made after covering these areas alone.

For a housewife, cleaning, shopping, cooking, political rallies, Women's Lib marches or some combination of these may constitute her work. A gambler may work at the track and the pool hall. In general, the work and school history answers the question "How do you spend your day?"

DRUGS AND ALCOHOL HISTORY

The therapist may find more resistance in questioning in these areas than in asking about work and school. The questions should be tailored to the patient and should generally be of the "How much do you?" type rather than the "Do you?" type. For example, a teenage "longhair" can be asked, "Do you smoke grass every day, or only occasionally?" You would ask a thirty-year-old lawyer, "Have you tried grass?" A 45-year-old housewife, "Do you use sleeping pills often or now and then?"

With young people it is productive to question in this fashion:

"Tell me about you and drugs"

"What do you mean, like grass?"

"Okay, how much do you smoke?"

"Oh, I guess about average."

"Is that pretty much every day?"

"When I can get it."

"Did you smoke this morning?"

"Yes, one joint."

"Does it do a good thing for you all the time?"

"I never got a really bad thing out of it, if that's what you mean."

"When is the last time you dropped acid?"

"About a month ago."

"Estimate how many trips you've taken."

"Oh, I forget."

"Well, would you say twenty, or a hundred or more?"

"Oh, I'd say about fifty."

"Over what period of time was that? A year or two?"

"More like three or four. I guess I trip about every month."

"How about mescaline?"

"Three or four times. That's harder to get."

"What other things have you gotten into?"

"Speed and pills. Cocaine a couple of times."

"Do you ever shoot anything?"

"Yes, I shot heroin once but I'm afraid of shooting. I don't want to mess my body up."

"Was the speed in pills or crystal?"

"Crystal. Snorted a couple of times. Never got strung out on it though. I've seen guys get really wasted on that stuff. Do you know that's more addicting than heroin?"

"Yes, I know. Have you ever gotten kind of hung up on anything?"

"Yes. About two years ago I was really into downs. You know, reds and barbs. Doridens too. Really screwed my head up. Used them to cool myself out but I got like lost in them. That's when I quit school. . . . "

Notice in this example how the patient warms up to the therapist, and how many other areas beside drugs open themselves up to further exploration. These other areas can be covered later in the interview. It is best to cover one area (like drugs) with one smooth sweep and then get the details in subsequent questioning. It would be nice to know how high the patient is now, after having "smoked" this morning, but this question could sound like an accusation if asked before the patient knows you. Later in the interview you can ask it gently. "You must have been worried about coming in here. Is that why you smoked this morning? Are you high now?" How about the acid trips? Fifty is a fairly high number. Some of them must have been "bummers." Ask him. He'll tell you. He likes you now. You can ask anything you want because he knows that you know what he is all about, and that makes him feel good.

The language in this interview was learned from patients, varies in different areas of the country and is constantly changing. If you don't know the street word for something, use the official name or ask the patient. When heroin addicts are talking about "skag," ask "what's skag?" They might laugh at your ignorance but you'll find out what it means. (In this case, who is dumb can be debated with them if you care to.) Don't ever use street words you read in a book, or of which you aren't sure. The use of street words only helps if it is done completely naturally.

Alcohol questioning should also be done of everyone and again tailored to each particular patient. A "longhair" is asked about wine, a husky college guy about beer, a housewife about cocktails, a businessman about alcohol and an alcoholic about booze. If your approach is wrong, the patient will tell you. When alcoholism is suspected, the whole range of questioning about the sequelae to the disease must be explored. Questions must be asked (in this case of both the patient and family) about binges, blackouts, amnesia, D.T.'s, morning drinking, solitary drinking, effect on work, arrests, physical condition, dietary habits, secret drinking and so forth. Once again, until you know this type of patient as a person and become thoroughly familiar with this life style, your questioning will have to be more formal. With experience it can be more intimate. Don't pretend to be familiar with something when you are a stranger to it.

Tell the patient you are a stranger and ask him to help show you around. (See Chapter 11, Drug Addiction and Alcoholism.)

SEX HISTORY

The sex life of a person is often the most sensitive barometer of changes in his emotional health. A manic person often finds the acute episode accompanied by hypersexuality. The neurotic person is often impotent or frigid. Some addictive persons go through a phase of addiction to sex, showing the same compulsive and ritualistic behavior toward sexual practices as toward the ritual of drug taking. Schizophrenics often find sex too confusing, frightening and intimate in the course of an acute episode and so return to masturbation during that time.

Society has certain formal attitudes about what is proper and what is improper sexual behavior. Almost everyone engages in some form that is "improper." About this they may feel guilty, embarrassed, proud, ashamed, blasé, defensive, peculiar or hostile.

In order to get into this area of a person's life the therapist must be secure about her own sexuality, and mature enough to be nonjudgmental yet have some understanding of the variety of sexual experiences.

It is rare to see destructive or bizarre sexuality in a community mental health center. Rapists, child molesters, exhibitionists, sado-masochists and other sexual psychopaths will be familiar to the nurse in a prison setting only. As mental health centers become interested in the prisoners deriving from their catchment area these matters may well become important to the community nurse. Questioning can safely avoid these exotic areas unless the patient volunteers something of this nature.

Whether they admit it or not people are (and for the history of the world have been) fascinated by and interested in knowing about the varieties of sexual expression. It is not possible to be interested in people and care about them without being curious about how they spend their day, what they like to do and what they do in bed. This curiosity is quite natural and human, but a professional mystique has developed that seems to require that doctors, nurses and teachers should somehow make their sexual curiosity disappear. We see no reason for professionals not to have it and in fact know of no way it can be made to go away. Furthermore, professionals from time to time find themselves sexually "turned on" by the people they serve. The nurse should be warned that such interest and innocent curiosity is viewed by many as prurient (dirty), voyeuristic (getting your jollies out of looking) and scatological (sexually filthy). These accusations can frighten and intimidate the student therapist who may actually feel something is wrong with her for *wanting* to know about a person's sex life and conclude that she is unprofessional if she finds herself viewing a patient with sexual interest. This is utter nonsense!

All of us have sexual feelings for patients whom we find particularly attractive. This is perfectly normal. It can even give a little burst of energy at the end of a hectic day. Being professional, however, demands that we keep the patient's concerns and the primary reason for his seeing us central to our thoughts and action. That's what we are paid for.

After establishing rapport through questioning about work, school, drugs, and alcohol the therapist may ask about sex, again tailoring it to the patient. The middle-aged depressed housewife can be asked "Have you noticed any change in your feelings about sex since you started feeling depressed?" The chances are great that she has. The young heavy drug taker can be asked "Do you have a sex life?" Chances are good he may not. If he says "Yes," ask "What does it consist of?" "How often do you have sex?" "Would you rather masturbate or have sex with another person?" The busy executive can be asked "Is sex a big part of your life?" It may not be.

During the questioning, anyone can be asked "Do you enjoy sex?" A lot of people don't. If that is the case, find out why they do it at all. They may say "Because my wife (husband) expects it" or "I get the urge and do it because the feelings bother me" or "It wouldn't be normal if I didn't, would it?"

Many patients will say "I have a normal sex life." Ask them what they mean. For some, intercourse once a month is normal (it is). For others, twice a day is normal (it is).

People use their hands, their mouths, their genitals and their ani in various combinations in normal sex. If the nurse is comfortable with this level of detail she will ask the questions in a comfortable way and get some very interesting answers. If she is not, she should stay with the more general questions above.

In the course of this portion of the interview the patient should be asked if he or she is homosexual or bisexual or has had any experiences of this sort, and whether there has been any experimentation or experience in group sex of any type or partner swapping (if the patient has a partner). Because nonverbal communication often shouts louder than spoken words, it is important for the nurse to be clear about her personal feelings (especially if they are strong feelings) whether she states them to the patient or not. For example, some persons in our society, for whatever reason, hate homosexuals and feel they are sick or disgusting or find them somehow threatening. Such persons may believe homosexuality to be like a cancer in our society, capable of destroying our youth, family structure, religion and our entire way of life. A prejudice that is this strong cannot be hidden. We consider it as irrational as the views people once held towards Protestants, Catholics, Jews, Communists and blacks at various times during our country's adolescence. The mental health professional with strong prejudical views about these or any other groups of people can do great harm to patients and rarely survives for long in the easy going atmosphere of a community mental health center.

Our view, shared by most of our colleagues in the field, is that homosexuality is a valid life style and not a sickness or a perversion. Occasionally homosexual people can be taught to act in a heterosexual way but this is rarely desirable. It is quite similar to teaching a left-handed person to write with his right hand. Both efforts tend to create more problems than they solve. On the other hand, the homosexual cannot be viewed as just being on the other side of the sexual coin, identical in all respects to the heterosexual. The homosexual grows up in a heterosexual family that is rarely cheerful about, and seldom accepting of, his sexual preference (if they know it). He often finds that his survival depends on being a loner or becoming a part of the homosexual subculture that has many of the characteristics of any other group that is alienated from and by the dominant society. He may flaunt his homosexuality in anger or conceal it in fear. It is not possible to be the object of man's inhumanity to man for very long without collecting some emotional problems, and most do in this situation. The problems, however, are not intrinsic to the fact of the patient's homosexuality but are the result of the attitude of the dominant society.

In addition, a homosexual person is also subject to the same genetic flaws, developmental traumas and emotional disabilities as a heterosexual person. It is usually due to these factors that all patients come to the center. The homosexual patient requires the same treatment for his depression or psychosis or whatever as anyone else plus all the support he can get to be himself in an often hostile environment. Society is getting more gentle—especially among the youth—but it still has a long way to go.

While estimates of the number of persons who have a "significant"* homosexual history varies from 10 to 20 percent of the general population, the majority of people have had "some" homosexual experiences, especially in adolescence, and sometimes later. The nurse should not give the impression from her attitude and questioning that she considers everyone with a homosexual history as "being" homosexual. They are not, any more than everyone with a heterosexual history is "necessarily" heterosexual.

When the nurse has either a fairly clear idea of what the patient's life is like within the parameters of work, drugs and sex, or has probed sufficiently to determine that she is not likely to find out during the first interview (seldom the case), she should sit back and consider for a moment the information that has been gathered.

Any questions that have not been covered should be gone over at this point. Details like medical history and family history can usually be gotten very quickly and easily. These formal matters are better left to the end when the patient knows you better, even though the write-up of the interview will be in reverse order.

When the nurse is satisfied that the interview is completed and has a fairly good idea about the diagnosis, prognosis and treatment plan,

---

*"Significant" means exclusive homosexuality or one or several years of predominantly homosexual activity.

the interview can be drawn to a close, giving the patient a little lead time to gather himself together. An average termination goes something like this: "We're going to have to quit in a few minutes, Mr. Jones. Are there any things we haven't covered or are there any questions you have at this point that I might answer for you?" If nothing further is forthcoming the therapist can ask "How are you feeling now?"

Some patients hold back a few embarrassing details until the very end and should be given the time to cover them. Some will want to know how *you* feel, or how you feel about them or whether you think they are "crazy" or whether they can be helped. These questions should be answered as completely as possible with the emphasis on your understanding of the patient and the healing process rather than the pathology. For example, "Well, it's clear to me how very worried and frightened you have been and I think your judgment was correct when you decided to come in for help. I expect that you already feel a little better (if that is the case; it usually is) and you have already taken the first step towards getting healthy again. I'm going to take you to the day hospital (or inpatient unit or outpatient department) where you will be going and show you around. Miss Brown is there. I think you'll like her. You'll also see Dr. Charles for medication. Is there anything else you want to go over before we leave?"

"WRITING UP" THE INTERVIEW

There are various formats for recording a psychiatric interview and all are acceptable. Some hospitals and mental health centers print outlines (see Mental Status Examination, Appendix I) to be filled in and some have computer forms for optical scanning called "automated psychiatric interview" forms. In the absence of these the nurse will have to write up her own. It should be a concise, formal, easy-to-read summary (in narrative or outline form) of her observations which anyone can quickly read yet which contains all of the important information that has been obtained. The following outline can serve as a guide:

I. Identifying Data. Name, age, sex, marital status, color, occupation.

Edwin Jones is a 33-year-old, black, male, unmarried storekeeper who has been unemployed for the past one-and-one-half years . . .

II. Chief Complaint: quote the patient if possible.

. . . he came voluntarily to the center because he has "trouble sleeping" and is "bothered by thoughts" . . .

III. Previous Psychiatric History

. . . His only previous treatment was at the age of 17 when he was admitted to the University Hospital for a "nervous breakdown." He was hospitalized for six weeks and received

chemotherapy (drug unknown) and psychotherapy which continued for seven months after he was discharged . . .

IV. Family History

. . . There is no known family history of mental disorder. Parents are living and well and brother age 35 is married and living in California . . .

V. Social History (work, school, drugs, sex, and parents and siblings)

. . . The patient dropped out of college (Middletown University) after completing two years—"it wasn't relevant," and went to work for his uncle who owns a chain of six neighborhood grocery stores. From age 23 to 31 he managed and operated one of these stores and was taken into partnership with his uncle six months before he suddenly stopped working. "I had too much to think about to bother with work." Patient reports having had an active sex life (heterosexual) until five years ago when he "lost interest." He always had a "few close friends" but hasn't "bothered" with them for several years and has spent his time at home "writing and thinking." He lives alone in a rented house. He denies ever having used drugs and drinks beer moderately (one to two quarts per week) . . .

VI. Medical History. Significant medical events, especially over past five years.

. . . The patient has had no medical treatment for other than the common cold for the past five years and claims "excellent physical health" . . .

VII. Mental Examination

A. General appearance, manner and attitude

. . . The patient is casually dressed but neat and clean. He is soft spoken and cooperative throughout the interview . . .

B. Thought life and mental trend

. . . The patient is preoccupied by religious thoughts and moral considerations, feeling he has a "mission" to make the world more loving. There is some blocking and occasional looseness of associations . . .

C. Affectivity and Mood

. . . The patient's affect seems appropriate to his thought content and somewhat blunted. His mood is concerned, thoughtful and somewhat worried.

D. Sensorium

1. Orientation: for time, place and person

. . . He is oriented in three spheres . . .

2. Consciousness

. . . and fully conscious and aware of his surroundings . .

3. Intelligence

. . . He appears to be of above average intelligence . . .

4. Conceptual, concrete and abstract thinking

. . . and is capable of both concrete and abstract thought . . .

5. Judgment and Insight

. . . His judgment appears somewhat impaired (he gave away his stereo to a man he had just met last week) and he has only minimal insight into the extent and nature of his illness. He is aware that "something is wrong" and appears motivated to follow through on treatment . . .

VIII. Diagnosis and Prognosis

. . . The diagnostic impression is "schizophrenic reaction, paranoid type" and the prognosis is considered good with therapeutic intervention . . .

IX. Disposition (treatment plan)

. . . Mr. Jones is considered an appropriate referral to Day Hospital and he agrees to begin there today. He should be started on medication at once. The doctor has been notified.

3

Formulating A
Diagnostic Impression

INTRODUCTION

The authors have no intention of presenting the various sides of the old argument as to whether nurses can or should interview, evaluate, diagnose and treat mentally ill patients. In the majority of community mental health centers they do any or all of these, depending on their training and skill. For the most part they are nurse specialists, practitioners or clinicians with a master's degree, but many have their bachelor's degree and extensive experience. That some centers and some psychiatrists are not open to this expanded nursing role goes without saying. The competent psychiatric nurse, however, will have no difficulty in finding a position in this field where she can enjoy a true colleague relationship with the psychiatrist. The nurse's written records of her observations and diagnostic impressions are legal documents and may be cited in court along with those of the psychiatrist.

Philosophy

The concordance rate in psychiatric diagnosis is amazingly low. Any five clinicians examining the same patient will tend to have at least three different diagnoses, and often will come up with five. "Diagnosis, even in the purely physical disorders, and with the aid of laboratory procedures, is not yet an exact science. Therefore, we cannot expect a high degree of accuracy with mental diseases. Standards of diagnosis may differ from state to state, and . . . the country as a whole."[1] Diagnosis in mental illness is an inexact science. Nevertheless, inexact as it may be as a science, psychiatric diagnosis is not only useful, it is absolutely necessary. The clinical classifications and nosological categories do offer the clinician an efficient and essentially reliable guide to the coding of major symptoms for the compilation of statistical data prerequisite to research and evaluation. Also, it is a descriptive, convenient and uniform (if imperfect) method of recording significant aspects of abnormal behavior and concomitant symptoms. Dr. Henry Brill, Chairman of the Committee on Nomenclature and Statistics (1960-65) for the American Psychiatric Association has succinctly stated the rationale for adhering to formal guidelines and categories in discussing and describing mental health problems:

> "Classification facilitates an orderly, cumulative recording of human experience, prepares the way and provides terms for generalized and abstract thinking, and is a preliminary step towards the manipulations of logic. The clinician must understand psychiatric classification if he is to understand the literature of psychiatry, much of which is recorded in nosological terms."[2]

The authors, despite a few misgivings about the still unresolved problems and issues of such classification, support the above statement. The fact is, as mental health professionals practicing in a community mental health center, we suggest it is not possible to eliminate the use of diagnostic categories and still communicate effectively with peers.

However, it might be more accurate if nurses, doctors, psychologists, social workers and other clinicians who are responsible for the evaluation and diagnosis of psychiatric patients give ground a little and label their labels for what they really are—diagnostic *impressions*.

Establishing A Diagnostic Impression

It has been said that neurotics build dream houses, but psychotics live in them.* This one-line summary of the psychiatric classification system, simplistic as it is, gives a clue as to how the labeling of patients is done. Minor distortions of reality, such as excessive fantasizing, inability to cope, and worrying, all lead the nosologist to consider the broader category of *neurotic illnesses* or *neuroses*. Major distortions of reality, such as hallucinations and delusions, massive withdrawal and major affective disturbances lead one to consider the *psychotic disorders* or *psychoses*.

The basic difference depends on how the patient perceives the world and people around him and how he handles (how he behaves with regard to) his perceptions. The full range of human behavior is continuous but has been divided into categories by common practice to make it easier to understand and to deal with. This should not be unfamiliar to the student. "Pure red" and "pure green" are regions of the continuous spectrum of color which we agree to label with those names. In nature, however, we see so many intermediate color values that we run out of names. There are an infinite number of possibilities. Ten different "red" flowers can come in ten different shades of red. Their common characteristic of "redness" consists of their being more or less at the red end of the spectrum, not in their being identical in

---

*. . . and psychiatrists collect the rent.

shade. When we look at a northern forest in the summer we all agree that it is green. We all see the subtle differences in shades of green and delight in them. We "know" that green is not blue. There are the trees, and there is the sky. However, when we try to classify the iridescent blue-green values in the wing of a butterfly we have problems, and so we hedge. We say "that spot is bluish-green or greenish-blue."

There are an infinite number of "steps" between the persons we see as suspicious and distrustful and those we see as having a frank paranoid psychosis. If they fall on the suspicious end of the spectrum we label them neurotic. On the other end we label them psychotic. If they fall in the middle we have a problem and so we hedge.

The first step in rational psychiatric diagnosis is to describe what we see, as discussed in "The Psychiatric Interview" (Chapter 2). Then we try to see if there is a label that describes that particular range of behavior. To do this we must know the "names of the primary colors" or the "notes of the scale." We must know the conventional psychiatric classification scheme which is in the DSM II, *Diagnostic and Statistical Manual of Mental Disorders,* Second edition.[3] (See Appendix II.)

Patients, being products of nature, have an irritating tendency to slide up and down the scale from day to day in the course of getting better or worse. Psychiatrists (for the same reason, we suppose) have an irritating tendency to make connections between the way the patient *appears* and the *cause* of the illness. This cannot be done. Nonetheless, DSM II is a hodgepodge of groupings, some based on how the patient looks and some based on supposed etiology. The student will have to bear with us, and it, and learn it. She should not get bogged down in it, however, and lose sight of the infinite variety in human expression and experience.

THE PSYCHOSES (THE MAJOR MENTAL ILLNESSES)

This classification includes those disorders which represent change and distortion in patterns of acting, thinking and feeling. Their chief characteristic is major deterioration in the functioning of the ego. The most commonly observed symptoms (one or several of which may appear) are:

1) Withdrawal from, or loss of contact with, reality (living in the "dream house").
2) Regression to a previous level of functioning (moving away from, instead of toward, maturity).
3) Distorted or inappropriate affect (emotional response).
4) Distortion in cognitive functioning (comprehension, judgment, reasoning, memory).
5) Deterioration of intellectual functioning (may be temporary in acute episodes or progressive in chronic cases.

It is usually irreversible in cases with a chronic organic basis for the psychosis).

6) Distortion in perception—illusions and hallucinations.°

7) Delusional content to thinking (may be delusions of grandeur, persecution, or reference).

8) Loss of, or reduction in, impulse control.

9) Marked interference in interpersonal relationships.

These symptoms rarely all appear at the same time and to the same degree. When that does occur, and it occasionally will, the patient is quite ill, whether acute or chronic.

Within the category of the psychoses, various subtypes show different groupings of these symptoms. Four symptom-clusters (diagnostic categories) under the psychoses to be discussed are:

1. Involutional psychosis.

2. Affective psychoses.

3. Schizophrenia.

4. Paranoid psychosis.

Involutional Psychosis

This disorder is generally first seen in patients over 45 years of age. It can be associated with menopause in the female, but it is seen just as frequently in men.

It is called a reactive psychosis, meaning that the symptoms are reactions to a change in life style and body function. Even without the presence of psychotic disintegration of the personality, many people in this "change-of-life" period experience some anxiety and depression due to the physical limitations and social restrictions of advanced age. Being old in our society°° is associated with being "finished," "washed-up," "worn-out," "over-the-hill" and generally on the decline.

SYMPTOMS

These include depression, fatigue, agitation, hypochondriasis, self-reproach, guilt, delusions of persecution (particularly in the paranoid types), and most characteristically a verbalized anxious anticipation of doom and disaster. Commonly such a patient will state, as he sits wringing his hands or pacing, "I feel like something awful is going to happen," and frequently there is an overall nihilistic flavor to the patient's language.

Chief differential diagnostic criteria are:

1. Age of the patient when first psychotic episode occurs (45-65).

°*Illusions* are false perceptions, like seeing a mirage in the desert; however they are real sensory experiences. *Delusions* are false beliefs, like the belief that one's body is turning to stone. *Hallucinations* are imaginary perceptions, like hearing voices when no one is there. They are not real sensory experiences.

°°This is not the case in other societies. (See Chapter 12, "The Older Adult.")

2. Absence of any organic symptoms. (See presenile psychoses, page 147.)

Affective Psychoses (Cyclothymic Reactions)

The chief characteristic of this group of reactions is mood swings which may range from profound depression to an acute manic episode, with periods of relative normality between psychotic episodes. Some patients experience both the manic and depressed phases cyclically but most just have recurrent depression or recurrent mania. (See Fig. 3-1.)

DEPRESSION
Early depression is characterized by mild psychomotor retardation and some preoccupation with suicidal ideas, with delusions and hallucinations being absent.* A later, or more severe, depression may show delusional ideation, feelings of doom and self-degradation, great concern about money and sin, anorexia with weight loss, constipation and insomnia. The possibility of suicidal gesture, or attempt, is real.

PROFOUND DEPRESSION
This is characterized by severe psychomotor retardation resulting in catatonic-like stupor. Such patients are usually unresponsive, mute and immobile; anorexia can result in extreme weight loss. When such symptoms are present, a thorough history should be taken from family or friends. Usually there will be some indication of past mood swings. Occasionally profoundly sick patients such as this are first seen on a home visit.

HYPOMANIA
This is difficult to assess because the patient generally feels so good that he rarely seeks psychiatric consultation unless he has had experience with similar episodes in the past and has been trained to monitor his own symptoms. Symptoms include a generalized expansiveness in affective response with uninhibited comments and behavior. An "anything goes" attitude seems to prevail, and initially there is an increased sense of well-being. As a rule there is an increased capacity for physical activity and such patients will describe their long and frequent walks, their sexual conquests and their lack of fatigue. Their judgment is impaired and becomes more so as the manic state increases.

ACUTE MANIC REACTION
This is the apogee of the affective psychoses, just as profound depression is the perigee. The patient's hypomania gradually or rapidly escalates to an irrational state. The symptoms usually include bizarre behavior and dress, rapid speech with loose associations, flight of ideas and delusions

---

*If this does not progress it should be classified under "psychoneurotic disorders."

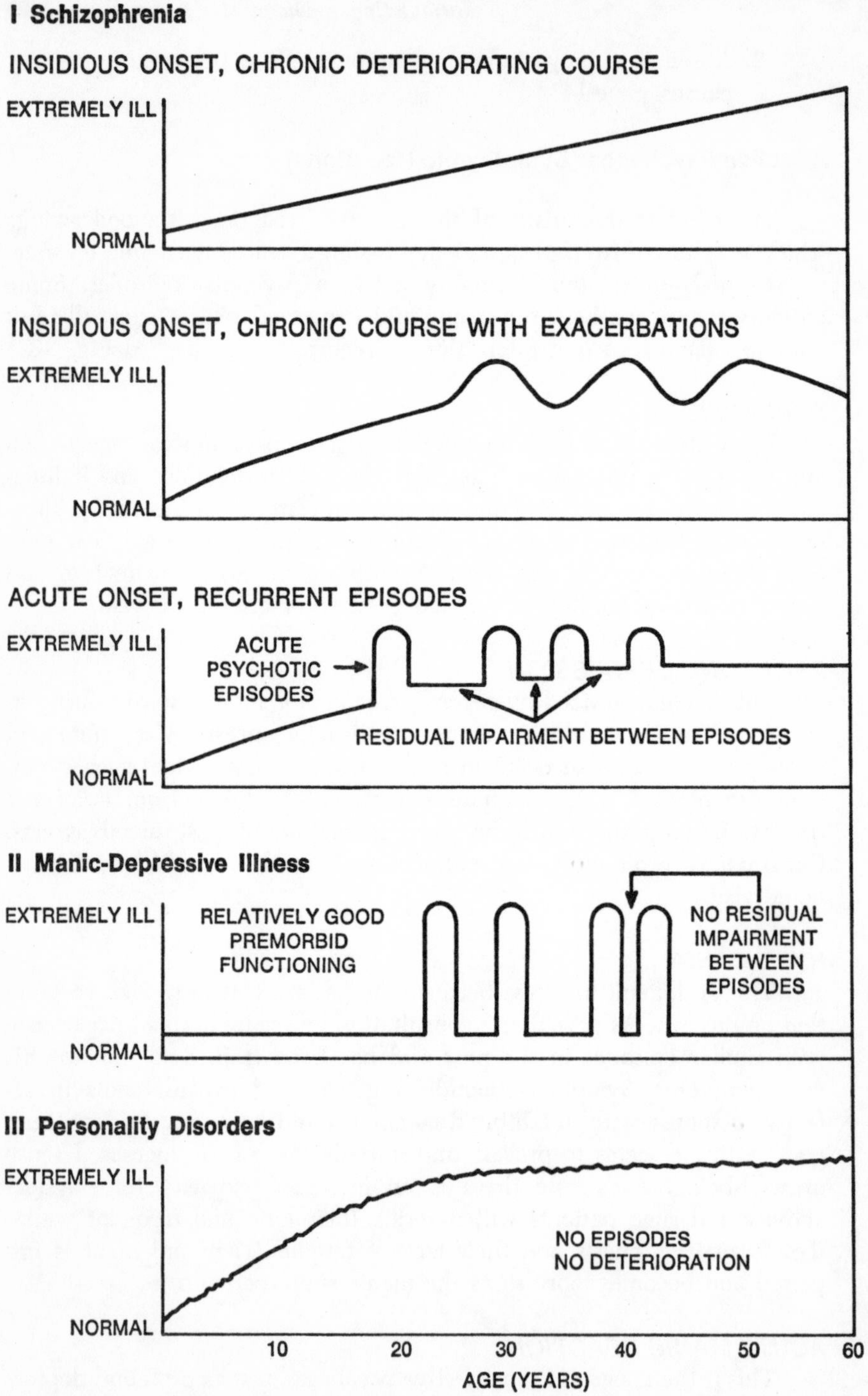

I Schizophrenia

INSIDIOUS ONSET, CHRONIC DETERIORATING COURSE

EXTREMELY ILL

NORMAL

INSIDIOUS ONSET, CHRONIC COURSE WITH EXACERBATIONS

EXTREMELY ILL

NORMAL

ACUTE ONSET, RECURRENT EPISODES

EXTREMELY ILL

ACUTE PSYCHOTIC EPISODES →

RESIDUAL IMPAIRMENT BETWEEN EPISODES

NORMAL

II Manic-Depressive Illness

EXTREMELY ILL

RELATIVELY GOOD PREMORBID FUNCTIONING

NO RESIDUAL IMPAIRMENT BETWEEN EPISODES

NORMAL

III Personality Disorders

EXTREMELY ILL

NO EPISODES NO DETERIORATION

NORMAL

10   20   30   40   50   60

AGE (YEARS)

Fig. 3-1. The typical courses of illness in schizophrenia contrast sharply with each other and with other disorders. (From Spitzer, R. L. and Endicott, Jean; Medcom ed. Schizophrenia: A Diagnostic Overview. New York: 1970.)

of grandeur. The uncontrolled symptoms can have tragic results if the patient is not treated. He frequently becomes involved in "deals," buying and selling anything, and/or spending life's savings at the drop of a hat. Families of such patients are usually frustrated, frightened, angry and exhausted in their efforts to manage and cope with the patient, and their descriptions of the patient's behavior as well as their reactions can assist in the diagnosis. Again, the most significant factor in formulating the diagnostic impression of an affective psychosis is the recurrent nature of the disorder, and the relative normality of the patient's life during the interim between psychotic episodes. (See Fig. 3-1.)

Schizophrenia (See Tables 3-1 and 3-2.)

Schizophrenia is the most prevalent of the psychotic disorders and probably the most feared psychiatric diagnosis. Frequently it is incorrectly assigned to patients because of the difficulty in accurate diagnosis. Any or all of the general symptoms of psychosis can be seen in schizophrenic reactions. Complicating the diagnostic picture is the fact that ". . . it is now well recognized that many patients for whom the diagnosis of schizophrenia is justified are not always in fact *functioning* at a psychotic level. This is particularly true in the early or convalescent stages of the illness."[4]*

The four classic and primary symptoms of schizophrenia are known as "the four A's":

1. Disturbances in *association* (loosened),
2. *Affect* (flattened),
3. *Ambivalence,* and
4. *Autism* (withdrawal from real world and preoccupation with idiosyncratic thoughts and fantasies).

---

*Here we get into the problem of diagnosis on the basis of suspected underlying *disease process* in addition to diagnosis on the basis of *symptom classes.*

TABLE 3–1—DIAGNOSTIC VALUE OF DIFFERENT SYMPTOMATOLOGY IN SCHIZOPHRENIA

Symptom	Definition	Diagnostic Weight
A. Symptomatology practically pathognomonic of schizophrenia. When present, the diagnosis is extremely likely.		
Flat effect	Generalized impoverishment of emotional reactivity. Impassive face, monotonous voice.	Very common in schizophrenia. Distinguish from a phasic condition in severe depression which the patient regards as pathological, shallow affect of organics and hysterics, and constricted affect of obsessional personality.

TABLE 3–1—(cont.)

Symptom	Definition	Diagnostic Weight
A. *(continued)*		
Thought disorder	Tendency of the associations to lose their continuity so that thinking becomes confused, bizarre, incorrect, and abrupt.	Very common in schizophrenia. Most diagnostic when found in a setting of clear consciousness. Distinguish from looseness of associations as found in manic states, and from dull intelligence and poor education.
Delusions of influence or passivity	Delusional belief that thoughts, moods, or actions are controlled or mysteriously influenced by other people or by strange forces.	Unusual in schizophrenia but present in no other condition.
Hallucinations of thoughts being broadcast or spoken aloud		Unusual in schizophrenia but present in no other condition.
Delusion that everyone knows what the patient is thinking		Unusual in schizophrenia but present in no other condition.
Specific catatonic symptoms Rigidity	Maintenance of a rigid posture against efforts to be moved.	Occasionally seen in schizophrenia, particularly during acute catatonic episodes or in regressed patients who have been hospitalized for many years. Similar behavior is sometimes associated with organic brain disease.
Waxy flexibility	Maintenance of postures (eg, if arm is raised, patient will leave it elevated).	
Posturing	Voluntary assumption of inappropriate or bizarre postures.	

B. Symptomatology seen in schizophrenia and rarely in other conditions. When present the diagnosis is very likely.

Apathy	Lack of feeling, interest, concern, or emotion.	Common in schizophrenia. Of diagnostic value only if not due to depressive syndrome.
Inappropriate affect	Affect which is incongruous in light of situation or content of thought.	Common in schizophrenia. Rule out manic, hysterical, or organic disorder.
Autism	Persistent tendency to withdraw from involvement with the external world and to become preoccupied with ideas and fantasies which are egocentric, illogical, and in which objective facts tend to be obscured, distorted, or excluded.	Common in schizophrenia. Rule out identification with a cultural subgroup which has deviant beliefs, as well as temporary withdrawal and preoccupation with fantasy life.

TABLE 3–1—(cont.)

Symptom	Definition	Diagnostic Weight
B. *(continued)*		
Catatonic stupor	Marked decrease in reactivity to environment and reduction of spontaneous movements and activity. Patient appears unaware of nature of surroundings, but generally is very aware.	Common in catatonic schizophrenics. Rule out organic brain disease, depressive disorder, or hysteria.
Neologisms	Invention of new words.	Unusual in schizophrenia but practically nonexistent in other conditions. Very suggestive of schizophrenia when accompanied by indifference to being understood.
Catatonic excitement	Apparently purposeless and stereotyped excited motor activity not influenced by external stimuli.	Rule out manic or hysterical excitement, which is more purposeful and responsive to external stimuli.
Bodily hallucinations	False sensory impression experienced in the body. Example: Patient feels electricity is being sent through him.	Rare in schizophrenia. Very diagnostic when associated with persecutory delusions.
Auditory hallucinations	False sensory impression of sound	Common in schizophrenia. Most diagnostic when voices. Unusual but present in affective psychoses and organic psychoses, particularly alcoholic hallucinosis.
C. Symptomatology commonly seen in schizophrenia and other conditions. When present the diagnosis is likely.		
Delusions	Conviction in some important personal belief which is almost certainly not true and is resistant to modification.	Rule out organic and other functional psychoses. In affective psychoses the content of the delusion is in harmony with the disordered mood. Bizarre, incomprehensible, or fragmentary delusions are more suggestive of schizophrenia.
Hallucinations	Sensory impression in the absence of external stimuli; occurs during the waking state.	Rule out organic and functional psychoses. When patient exhibits an inadequate emotional reaction, it suggests schizophrenia.
Inappropriate or bizarre behavior	Behavior that is odd, eccentric, or not in keeping with the situation.	Rule out organic and functional psychoses. The more incomprehensible the behavior, the more likely is schizophrenia.
Extreme social isolation	Avoidance of contact or involvement with people	Also common in alcoholism, schizoid personality, and depressive illnesses.

TABLE 3–1—(cont.)

Symptom	Definition	Diagnostic Weight
C. *(continued)*		
Markedly unstable interpersonal relationships	Relationships with relatives, friends, and associates tend to be stormy and ambivalent. Minor difficulties lead to anger and disruption of the relationship.	Also common in hysterical and paranoid personalities. The more chaotic the history of relationships, the more suggestive of schizophrenia.
Ideas of reference	Detection of personal reference in seemingly insignificant remarks, objects, or events. May be of sufficient intensity to be a delusion. Example: Patient interprets a person's sneeze as a message.	Rule out other psychoses. Occasionally seen in suspicious people who are not otherwise psychotic.
Poor academic and occupational adjustment		Present in all other conditions. Is more suggestive of schizophrenia when variable over period of time and there is a marked discrepancy between level of functioning and background or previous achievements.
Excessive concern with body symptoms	Includes preoccupation with real or imagined physical appearance, fears of becoming ill; health rituals.	Rule out depressive illness and hypochondriacal neurosis. Bizarre or incomprehensible complaints or beliefs are suggestive of schizophrenia.

TABLE 3–2—MAJOR DIFFERENTIAL DIAGNOSES OF SCHIZOPHRENIA SUBTYPES

SCHIZOPHRENIA SUBTYPE	DIFFERENTIAL DIAGNOSIS
Paranoid	1. Involutional paranoid state 2. Paranoia 3. Amphetamine-toxic psychosis 4. Paranoid personality
Simple	1. Schizoid personality
Childhood	1. Behavior disorders of childhood and adolescence 2. Withdrawing reaction
Schizoaffective	1. Manic-depressive, manic 2. Psychotic depression 3. Cyclothymic personality
Latent	1. Severe neurosis 2. Severe personality disorder
Catatonic	1. Retarded depression
Chronic undifferentiated	1. Chronic organic brain syndrome 2. Chronic use of stimulants or hallucinogens
Acute schizophrenic episode	1. Severe transient situational disturbance 2. Acute organic brain syndrome

Tables 3-1 and 3-2 reprinted with permission from Spitzer, R. L., and Endicott, J.: "Schizophrenia: A Diagnostic Overview." *In* Medcom, Inc. (eds.), Schizophrenia. New York: J. B. Roerig, 1970.

SCHIZOPHRENIA SUBTYPES

There are ten subgroupings under the schizophrenia classification of psychosis. The authors have utilized the descriptions given in the DSM II.[5] (See Table 3-3.) The code numbers designated to the left of each subtype are used for much the same reason as library codes—to organize and simplify classification. The hues in the schizophrenic spectrum frequently blend with each other and often look different to observers, depending on the light.

TABLE 3–3—SCHIZOPHRENIC SUBTYPES

295.0 Schizophrenia, simple type	This psychosis is characterized chiefly by a slow and insidious reduction of external attachments and interests and by apathy and indifference leading to impoverishment of interpersonal relations, mental deterioration, and adjustment on a lower level of functioning. In general, the condition is less dramatically psychotic than are the hebephrenic, catatonic, and paranoid types of schizophrenia. Also, it contrasts with schizoid personality, in which there is little or no progression of the disorder.
295.1 Schizophrenia, hebephrenic type	This psychosis is characterized by disorganized thinking, shallow and inappropriate affect, unpredictable giggling, silly and regressive behavior and mannerisms, and frequent hypochondriacal complaints. Delusions and hallucinations, if present, are transient and not well organized.
295.2 Schizophrenia, catatonic type 295.23 *Schizophrenia, catatonic type, excited* 295.24 *Schizophrenia, catatonic type, withdrawn*	It is frequently possible and useful to distinguish two subtypes of catatonic schizophrenia. One is marked by excessive and sometimes violent motor activity and excitement and the other by generalized inhibition manifested by stupor, mutism, negativism, or waxy flexibility. In time, some cases deteriorate to a vegetative state.
295.3 Schizophrenia, paranoid type	This type of schizophrenia is characterized primarily by the presence of persecutory or grandiose delusions, often associated with hallucinations. Excessive religiosity is sometimes seen. The patient's attitude is frequently hostile and aggressive, and his behavior tends to be consistent with his delusions. In general the disorder does not manifest the gross personality disorganization of the hebephrenic and catatonic types, perhaps because the patient uses the mechanism of projection, which ascribes to others characteristics he cannot accept in himself. Three subtypes of the disorder may sometimes be differentiated, depending on the predominant symptoms: hostile, grandiose, and hallucinatory.
295.4 Acute schizophrenic episode	This diagnosis does not apply to acute episodes of schizophrenic disorders described elsewhere. This condition is distinguished by the acute onset of schizophrenic symptoms, often associated with confusion, perplexity, ideas of reference, emotional turmoil, dreamlike dissociation, and excitement, depression, or fear. The acute onset distinguishes this condition from simple schizophrenia. In time these patients may take on the characteristics of catatonic, hebephrenic, or paranoid schizophrenia, in which case their diagnosis should be changed accordingly. In many cases the patient recovers within weeks, but sometimes his disorganization becomes progressive. More frequently remission is followed by recurrence.

TABLE 3–3—(cont.)

295.5 Schizophrenia, latent type	This category is for patients having clear symptoms of schizophrenia but no history of a psychotic schizophrenic episode. Disorders sometimes designated as incipient, prepsychotic, pseudoneurotic, pseudopsychopathic, or borderline schizophrenia are categorized here.
295.6 Schizophrenia, residual type	This category is for patients showing signs of schizophrenia but who, following a psychotic schizophrenic episode, are no longer psychotic.

295.7 Schizophrenia, schizoaffective type	This category is for patients showing a mixture of schizophrenic symptoms and pronounced elation or depression. Within this category it may be useful to distinguish excited from depressed types as follows:
	    295.73 Schizophrenia, schizoaffective type, excited
	    295.74 Schizophrenia, schizoaffective type, depressed

295.8 Schizophrenia, childhood type	This category is for cases in which schizophrenic symptoms appear before puberty. The condition may be manifested by autistic, atypical, and withdrawn behavior; failure to develop identity separate from the mother's; and general unevenness, gross immaturity, and inadequacy in development. These developmental defects may result in mental retardation, which should also be diagnosed.
295.9 Schizophrenia, chronic undifferentiated type	This category is for patients who show mixed schizophrenic symptoms and who present definite schizophrenic thought, affect, and behavior not classifiable under the other types of schizophrenia. It is distinguished from schizoid personality.

Source: Diagnostic and Statistical Manual of Mental Disorders, 2nd edition. Washington, D. C.: The American Psychiatric Association, 1968.

Paranoid Psychoses

Patients in this psychotic grouping have a concrete and pervasive delusional system which is generally persecutory. They make extensive use of the mental mechanism of projection and their delusions are not perceived by themselves as pathological. They are not likely to seek psychiatric consultation, and are usually tolerated as "the neighborhood crank" in their communities. They are chronically suspicious, distrusting most people, distant but not withdrawn and have very poor insight. In areas outside of their delusional system they retain good contact with reality. The paranoid patient is suspicious in the interview situation and may play a cat-and-mouse game in giving historical data and insist on asking the questions. The paranoid person frequently has a "pseudo-community" in his head, referred to as "them" which is "an imaginary organization composed of real and imagined persons, whom the patient represents as united for the purpose of carrying out some action upon him."[6] It is often difficult to distinguish between a paranoid psychosis and paranoid schizophrenia.

PSYCHONEUROTIC DISORDERS (The Minor Mental Illnesses)

As compared to patients with psychoses, those suffering from neuroses:

1) Correctly interpret external reality (no delusions or hallucinations)
2) Remain in contact with reality
3) Exhibit ego integration and personality organization.

The symptoms of most psychoneurotic disorders present as exaggerations of normal behavior.

For the beginning clinician it is more difficult to be accurate in the diagnosis of neurotic than psychotic disorders. One factor in this difficulty is the natural, but rarely mentioned, reaction of the novice clinician to the patient's recitation of his symptoms. The clinician tends to think "Hmm—that's not too bad, I do that myself," or. "I never did that! This patient must be sick." Such identification of the clinician with the symptoms that neurotic patients present makes objectivity difficult. However, this situation improves with increased experience.

The core symptom of the neuroses is anxiety. Anxiety is a warning that the ego is having difficulty in its role of satisfying the demands of the superego, the id and the outside world. A compromise cannot be struck and something must give.

The neurotic patient is engaged in a conflict with which he cannot cope. Rarely is the conflict clearly visible to the patient at first, since most of it occurs in the unconscious. It is not necessary in most cases, however, for the conflict to be eased out of the patient's mind and held up for examination in psychoanalysis in order to relieve the anxiety. (See Chapter 5, "Psychotherapy.") Anxiety is the dynamic center of neuroses, may not always be expressed directly, and may be converted, displaced or camouflaged. However, the patient is acutely aware of a sense of discomfort regardless of the unconscious attempt to control or modify it. Physical symptoms commonly experienced are muscular tension, headaches, gastro-intestinal upsets, excessive perspiration and sighing respiration.

The subtypes are listed in the DSM II. We will only discuss here those neuroses encountered most frequently in a community mental health setting. Not mentioned are the infrequently seen neurasthenia, hypochondriasis, and depersonalization syndromes. Patients with some of the symptoms characteristic of these disorders are seen, but generally the symptoms of extreme fatigue and exhaustion (neurasthenia), preoccupation with body function and fear of disease (hypochondriasis), and estrangement from self, body or surroundings (depersonalization) occur in relationship to the neurotic disorders we describe rather than as discrete diagnostic patterns.

Under psychoneurotic disorders we include:

1) Anxiety neurosis

2) Hysterical neurosis (conversion reaction)
3) Phobic reactions
4) Obsessive compulsive neurosis
5) Depressive neurosis.

Anxiety Neurosis

This is frequently manifested by the patient's excessive and un-realistic concern with almost any situation. There may be somatic symptoms, difficulty in breathing and chest pain, without physiologic cause. Such patients may present symptoms of extreme fearfulness bordering on panic. Characteristically, there is no real and present danger to the patient. The disorder may have an acute or gradual onset which eventually becomes chronic.

Hysterical Neurosis (Conversion Reaction)

This disorder is usually seen as a dramatic physical response due to unacceptable unconscious impulses being converted into bodily symptoms. It may follow a traumatic event or emotionally charged situation in the patient's life. Such patients can report sudden loss of function resulting in paralysis, blindness, or deafness. These patients are frequently impulsive, immature, dependent and attention-seeking. Differential diagnosis to rule out any organic basis for the loss of body function is essential. Significantly, these patients do not seem to demonstrate appropriate concern over their loss of function and may seem gratified by the resultant attention paid them.

Phobic Reactions

Patients suffering from this disorder complain of unreasonable fear and apprehension about an object, person, or situation which they can identify as having no real foundation. It is severe enough at times to make them prisoners in their own homes and usually is a maladaptive attempt to avoid anxiety-producing situations. There are often physical manifestations of the extreme apprehension they experience, such as palpitations, perspiration, nausea and tremors. Examples of phobias are fear of heights, open spaces and dirt.

Obsessive Compulsive Neurosis

The main symptom presented in this disorder is the insistent, repetitive intrusion of ideas, thoughts, impulses and actions which the patient is unable to control. Generally, the patient is aware that the behavior is unreasonable, and there is impatience with the impairment of adaptive functioning due to the symptoms. The patient may feel compelled to carry out ritualistic handwashing, touching or counting.

Depressive Neurosis

This disorder is essentially an *over*reaction or protracted reaction to the genuine loss of a treasured possession or loved one. Common symptoms include sadness, frequent crying, moderate anorexia and weight loss, mild and transient disturbance in sleep patterns and fatigue.

THE PERSONALITY DISORDERS

Patients with personality disorders show patterns of chronic, life-long maladaptive behavior and occasionally exhibit symptoms suggestive of psychotic or psychoneurotic disorders. They can be distinguished from the psychotic disorders by their lack of ego disintegration and diffusion resulting in impaired reality testing, and thought disorder. They can be differentiated from the psychoneurotic disorders because neurotic patients remain capable of maintaining some level of rationality in interpersonal relations; whereas, patients with personality disorders often have great difficulty relating to others. The general symptoms of the personality disorders include one or several of the following:

1. Poor interpersonal relationships
2. Inability to feel or experience emotion (they are sometimes accurately described as "cold and unfeeling")
3. Poor concentration
4. Poor motivation
5. Reluctance to accept rules and regulations
6. Poor judgment
7. Minimal insight
8. Poor impulse control.

The majority of patients who suffer from personality disorders are able to adjust marginally and do not engage in serious criminal acts. However, their defective personalities predispose them to a disregard for accepted social behavior.

Community mental health centers located in densely populated urban areas probably have more frequent contact with such patients than do smaller centers in rural areas. This is so because the largeness and impersonal nature of urban areas offer greater anonymity and tolerance of peculiar behavior. When these individuals seek psychiatric consultation, as they frequently do, careful attention should be paid to their previous psychiatric contacts. It is not unusual to find one or more active involvements with other community mental health centers in the same area. The initial evaluation of one of these patients can be trying but the nurse will be most effective if she can retain control of the interview session, despite attempts by the patient to provoke and manipulate.

Under personality disorders we include the following subtypes most frequently seen in community mental health center practice:
1) Paranoid personality
2) Cyclothymic personality
3) Schizoid personality
4) Explosive personality
5) Obsessive compulsive personality
6) Hysterical personality
7) Antisocial personality.

Paranoid Personality

Marked suspiciousness in the absence of a delusional system is the chief characteristic of this disorder. Additional symptoms include distrust, jealousy and envy, hostility, excessive utilization of projection (with inferred slights and ruminations about revenge which are occasionally verbalized during the intake interview). Such patients naturally tend to be loners. They are simply unable to trust or tolerate the intimacy of close relationships.

Cyclothymic Personality

Mood swings with no impairment in reality testing or cognition are characteristic of this disorder. The affect is labile and the patient will experience chronic highs and lows unless the symptoms can be resolved.

Schizoid Personality

This is very similar in manifest symptoms to the simple schizophrenic subtype. There is shyness, seclusiveness, poverty of interpersonal relationships, and egocentric or autistic thinking *without* impairment in reality testing. A significant distinction between this disorder and schizophrenia is its static quality. Untreated there is little remission or progression of the process.

Explosive Personality

Sudden violent outbursts of rage with little or no external provocation is characteristic of this disorder. Although the patient may be remorseful after the outburst he is unable to control the verbal or physical aggressiveness which is chronic and recurrent.

Obsessive Compulsive Personality

This disorder is characterized by overconcern with detail, rigidity, indecision and doubt, inhibitions and moralistic excess. Such patients present as the "holier-than-thou," "uptight," "can't-make-up-my-mind" type.

Hysterical Personality

Symptoms differ from hysterical neurosis in that psychogenic loss or disorder of function is not observed. These patients are immature, dependent, self-dramatizing (histrionic), impulsive, seductive and susceptible to suggestion. They usually demand (and are accustomed to receiving) lots of attention and will "act out" in order to receive it.

Antisocial Personality

As a group, these patients probably cause the most problems in society. They have frequently been in difficulty with the law, and might first be seen in psychiatric consultation on the recommendation of the court or probation office. They are unable to tolerate frustration, are easily enraged and can act out violently without feeling remorseful. They will sometimes describe themselves as "cold-blooded," and are often described by others as such. They can be ruthless and vindictive and tend to blame others for their behavior.

The student should not assume that all persons having a past record of law-breaking are antisocial personalities.

SITUATIONAL DISORDERS

So far in this chapter we have emphasized diagnosis on the basis of symptom clusters and avoided, where possible, discussion of etiology and theoretical constructs. This is in keeping with our purpose of providing the nurse with practical information that will be immediately useful in her day-to-day functioning in a community mental health center.

There are other mental health disturbances the nurse will be called upon to evaluate which have not been described. These include non-psychotic disorders which are situational and are classified under transient situational disturbances; they include the adjustment reactions of adolescence, adult life and old age. In these conditions the reaction is to overwhelming environmental stress, and the patient may present acute symptoms of varying severity but will reconstitute quickly with direct supportive intervention. One would expect the community mental health nurse to see many such cases because of the environmental stress which is endemic in the sprawling urban areas where most centers are located. However, it is seen only infrequently.

TREATMENT PLAN

It is the responsibility of the nurse who has interviewed and carefully assessed the patient to formulate a treatment plan based on her impressions of the patient's need for treatment and the nurse's knowledge of available resources. Some patients can wait while others cannot. It is the task of the nurse making this judgment to consider the effect of delay in treatment on an individual basis. If the decision is to be referral to outpatient for individual therapy and the nurse making the referral knows that this would involve a waiting period of several weeks, she must be reasonably certain that the patient can tolerate the delay. This skill is developed with experience.

However, there is data available which can be helpful to the nurse as she makes her decision. The nurse must make it a point to be familiar with the therapeutic programs and style of the various units and therapists in the community mental health center, which are often quite varied. Likewise, the nurse should also get to know other community agencies and the services they can and cannot provide, for example, their fees and admission criteria. To write the name of another agency on a piece of paper and suggest to the patient that *he* contact the agency is to be unaware of the great effort most patients make to initiate and follow-through with their *first* contact.

Furthermore, it is insensitive to the constant hassles of those who seek clinic services because that is all they can afford or "are entitled to." The forms, questions, statements and processing that so many agencies (including community mental health centers) require of the clients or patients they serve often detract from whatever service they are trying to provide.

To facilitate the making of a suitable and responsive case disposition, the following considerations may assist the inexperienced nurse in establishing criteria for a decision:

1. *Formulation of a priority system,* reflecting symptom type and severity and the margin of safety for treatment delay.
2. *Availability of treatment modality,* including other resources, if necessary.
3. *Length of waiting list,* if any, for treatment of choice.
4. *Interim treatment plans and options,* when delay in treatment of choice is likely. (This may include plans for interim contact by phone or in person with the intake interviewer, or it may include referral to a "holding group" —open-ended therapy or medication group for waiting patients.)
5. *Motivational factors,* including patient's interest in, and desire for, treatment. An assessment of the likelihood of "follow-through" or "drop-out."
6. *Ability of patient* to consent to treatment (minors may need parental consent).
7. *Social factors,* including ability or inability to pay for treatment.* Attention should be paid to other agency involve-

---

*In some states welfare patients are able to receive any degree of service or treatment, with temporal limits in a given period, *without fee,* while marginal income patients must be able to pay for any and all treatment unless they are willing to file a declaration of poverty.

ment to avoid duplication of service or to arrange for additional services.

8. *Medical factors* should be considered and medical consultation should be sought if there is any suggestion of organic disease or malfunction.

It is a good idea to discuss a case with a colleague before making a disposition whenever possible. When there is uncertainty about the accuracy of the diagnosis or appropriateness of the disposition, consultation should be arranged with either a more experienced peer or preceptor. Occasionally the consultation will include another interview and the patient's fears about the significance of such a procedure should be considered.

The decision to interview the patient's spouse, parents or entire family as a further aid in deciding both the diagnosis and disposition must also be considered. The rationale for this move should be explained: "I'd like to talk to your wife, Mr. Jones, to get a better idea of the situation." In such instances the apprehension, if there is any, is likely to be the wife's as she tries to designate her husband as the real and only patient.

Naturally, the techniques in interviewing, differentiating and weighing symptoms, classifying pathology, establishing a diagnosis and formulating a treatment plan and case disposition are skills the inexperienced nurse will need to develop. As in most things, experience is the best teacher—but in mental health practice a solid theoretical base helps too.

REFERENCES

1. Malzberg, Benjamin. "Important Statistical Data About Mental Illness." *In* S. Arieti (ed.), American Handbook of Psychiatry. New York: Basic Books, 1959. p. 164.
2. Brill, Henry. "Classification and Nomenclature of Psychiatric Conditions." *In* S. Arieti (ed.), American Handbook of Psychiatry. New York: Basic Books, 1966. p. 5.
3. Diagnostic and Statistical Manual of Mental Disorders, 2nd edition. Washington, D. C.: American Psychiatric Association, 1968.
4. Spitzer, R. L. and Endicott, J. "Schizophrenia: A Diagnostic Overview." *In* Medcom, Inc. (eds.), Schizophrenia. New York: J. B. Roerig, 1970. p. 9.
5. Diagnostic and Statistical Manual of Mental Disorders, 2nd edition. Washington, D. C.: The American Psychiatric Association, 1968.
6. Cameron, N. "Paranoid Conditions and Paranoia." *In* S. Arieti (ed.), American Handbook of Psychiatry. New York: Basic Books, 1966. p. 518.

4
Crisis Intervention

As in so many areas of psychiatric treatment the name of the specific therapy is new, but little else. Crisis intervention of some type has been going on since people began interacting with and reacting to each other and their environment; they just didn't know what to call it. Today we do, and in addition to giving it a name, we have developed a wider understanding of what a crisis is, what factors contribute to its cause and why individuals react the way they do in crisis situations. We have a theory and an understanding of the psychodynamics involved. The development of a specific technique to assist people who are experiencing crisis has been built upon the less formal but effective ways with which such situations were dealt in the past.

The formal explication of a crisis theory is fairly recent. In the early 1940's Lindemann reported and commented on his observations of the crisis response many people had to their involvement in the Cocoanut Grove fire in Boston, in which hundreds of people lost their lives.[1] His observations and theoretical suggestions were widely hailed as significant in understanding what people do when faced with emergency situations. Later, the experience of many psychiatrists responsible for the examination and treatment of battle-weary, frightened and disturbed soldiers during World War II and the Korean War was also reported. Together these studies could probably be cited as the keystone of the formal development of crisis theory.

Crisis theory is a significant development in modern psychiatric thought because it represents a shift in focus from the psyche in the individual to the individual in his environment, and de-emphasizes the feeling that intrapsychic aspects of the individual psyche are the most important considerations in mental disorder. There is, finally, recognition of the social milieu and its structure as contributing factors in both the development of an individual's psychiatric symptoms (in response to a crisis situation) and his recovery. This seems to us so necessary and logical a consideration that it is difficult to comprehend how radical a departure such theory represents from the basic psychoanalytic and psychodynamic formulations of the Freudians and early neo-Freudians.

Given the increasing pressures and exigencies of urban life, particularly those of the inner city where for many life at times seems to consist of hurdling one crisis after another, it is likely that crisis theory would have inevitably developed. When "coping" becomes almost synonymous with functioning, as it has for many people in our society today, then crisis theory and intervention techniques are necessary tools of the trade for any community mental health nurse.

SOME COMMENTS ON CRISIS THEORY

The word crisis has as its root the Greek word *krinein* which means "to decide." Decision—the reluctance, resistance, or inability to make it— is probably the most characteristic aspect of a crisis. Crises are turning points, points of change, junctures; they are climactical and they involve the use of judgment. "Crises are the crucibles out of which many innovations emerge; new modes of action often receive their initial direction from attempts to cope with emergencies."[2] The crisis situation, when successfully negotiated, generally leads to continued maturation and development. A crisis arises, past coping measures are tried unsuccessfully, new measures evolve, are adapted, the crisis is met, it abates and the individual experiences enhanced self-image because he has "met the crisis." In contrast, the individual faced with a crisis but unable to make a decision experiences increased anxiety and stress (always inherent in crisis situations). This stress, if not handled adequately, may lead to exacerbation of earlier and previously latent psychological conflicts. The crisis now becomes more complex and stressful. Resolution seems less possible to the individual. What is happening is that the emergence of previously latent conflicts now contributes to the dimension and shape of the crisis, generating new conflicts, and gives rise to a repetitive series of symptoms that psychological theory holds to be a characteristic of all neuroses. It is frequently at this point that the individual, or a member of his family, seeks advice and the process of crisis intervention begins. (Let us make a distinction between an emergency and a crisis—they are not identical. An emergency is a situational threat; it becomes a crisis when the person who is faced with the threat becomes anxious and begins to explore his capacity to do something about it.) Now, the significance of seeking help during a crisis is this: persons seeking resolution of crisis situations are more amenable to altering old and unsuccessful coping mechanisms and are most likely to succeed in learning new and more functional and adaptive behavior when the crisis intervention is provided by a skilled person. The duration of such intervention is brief; crises, according to crisis theory, have temporal limitations.

There are two broad categories of crises according to psychological theory:

1. Developmental Crises

These are critical transition points, which are universal—birth, adolescence, marriage, aging and death. Erikson has written of eight developmental stages, and postulates (with the support of both historians and anthropologists) that these exist in all cultures and always have.[3] Crises which arise in relation to this developmental construct are generally more personal, and because of the increasing urbanization and secularization, particularly as we see it in American inner cities today, these crises are more traumatic experiences than they have been in the past.

2. Coincidental Crises

These are crises which occur at random times in most of our lives. They include: accidents, including those which are near fatal; life-threatening experiences, such as war, natural disasters, earthquakes, fires, and floods; physical and mental illness; and those stresses related to the loss of income, prestige, status, job security, relocation, and immigration. (We can all think of personal examples in our own lives, including those common crises we shared as a nation during the 1963 missile crisis, the political assassinations of the 1960's, and, going back to the 1930's, the depression.)

Each individual develops a state of emotional, social, physiologic, and neurologic equilibrium which, although similar to others, is essentially as unique for that individual as his fingerprints. Such development is characteristic of normal maturation and is responsible for regulating the evenness of our responses, both physically and emotionally, to internal and external stimuli; it keeps us "on an even keel." Sometimes we speak of this stabilizing force as homeostasis, even though its success can be measured by its dynamic rather than static quality. After all, normal, individual functioning is not static; it allows for a variety of responses. It changes day by day as situations or input change. We react, in normal functioning, to preserve and maintain optimal levels of metabolic and psychologic function.

That some people are happier than others, have greater ups and downs, are more successful, are more or less effective than other people, are all characteristics of their individual, normal homeostasis. But, in the long run, despite the fluctuations in response, a picture unique to each individual becomes apparent: his way of dealing with problems, his highs and lows, his way of reacting to stress and pressure, his susceptibility or resistance to physical illness. All these responses differ from individual to individual, although there are sufficient similarities for us to establish norms of response to cover most situations, or to predict with some acuracy how a person or group of persons would react in a given unfamiliar situation. In a more specific way, this picture makes it easier for us to get along with those closest to us—parents, peers, siblings, colleagues, teachers, spouses—because its pattern becomes so familiar. However, this holds true for only as long as the environment is the same or predictable. Imagine, for example, how totally alien and devastating the environment must have been for the people of Hiroshima and Nagasaki when the atomic bombs fell on their cities. The quality of their crisis probably cannot be measured. But the astronauts, despite the alien environment of the moon, could survive, and effectively, because they were able to predict much of what they would experience and encounter.

Much of crisis theory concerns a person's ability to cope or to solve problems. Caplan has postulated that in normal functioning man daily encounters situations which can be successfully negotiated, using familiar techniques to maintain homeostasis. Success in reestablishing equilibrium depends on the organism's ability to counterbalance the opposing force; this is accomplished unconsciously or automatically by the mind and the body.[4] We know that the physical response is automatic, controlled by the autonomic nervous system responding instantaneously to change in environment. It is not difficult to imagine that the unconscious mind can similarly respond to change. But, when a crisis situation introduces stimuli which the individual using past techniques of problem solving is unable to deal with effectively—anxiety results. The problem remains unsolved; it doesn't go away. The integrity of the physical or intrapsychic system is threatened and anxiety increases. The individual's repertory of suitable or successful responses is depleted and now, in desperation, he "grasps at straws" or will try anything to solve the problem, maintain homeostatic integrity and reduce anxiety.

Sometimes, in these radical efforts to cope, the person succeeds, and, in doing so, realizes increased physical or emotional strength. When it happens that an individual succeeds in the face of overwhelming odds he frequently becomes a hero. Some people, in reaction to this phenomenon, deliberately place themselves in crisis situations to win handsome awards or accolades (e.g., students who compete for first place, businessmen who go after the big job, athletes who try for the big win) and if the situation is sufficiently critical or dangerous then a place in history is the reward. Charles "Lucky Lindy" Lindbergh is one example.

Our society places much value on the qualities of mental and physical endurance. In a sense, this love affair with success has added a burden on many Americans as they attempt to "measure up." Think of the subtle pressures we are all subjected to on a daily basis. We must look attractive and be physically fit, we must persevere and succeed, we must sacrifice and enjoy it, we must be competitive and win. Look at our slogans: "Scouting builds men," "The Army builds character." Our preoccupation with the symbols of success reveals much about us and our values and predisposes some of us to emotional and physical crises as we try to accomplish with ease, grace and style the "ideals" which may remain elusive.

When success in problem solving fails, after anxiety and tension have produced our last supereffort, the result will be regression to a lower, safer, more comfortable level of functioning. We all experience this regression at one time or another; it is characterized by the face-saving response "it really wasn't *that* important." But, if the situation is loaded (and that is a qualitative appraisal which differs for each individual), then the odds increase. In some ways the seriousness of the crisis which develops when a situation cannot be resolved successfully can be predicted by the value the individual places on winning, or at least avoiding failure. A good example is the soldier going into battle; it's a crisis because if he makes a mistake, or is unlucky, he is likely to die.

When the problem is profound and persists over a period of days or weeks without resolution, the crisis can provoke an emotional reaction which, depending on the individual's personality and investment in the situation, is characterized at least by regression and at worst by personality disorganization and distortion. The response is in part based on the individual's investment in the problem he can't solve, and his personality integration and adaptability before the crisis.

Crises have temporal limitations—they don't go on and on. They can't. People, no matter how well adapted or integrated, cannot survive the enormous levels of anxiety and tension a serious crisis generates. They must solve the problem, cope with it, regress, or "crack up" because of it, but one way or the other, it is not a static condition. This is important for the nurse, or any clinician, to know. The rapidity with which the crisis reaction moves demands immediate and skillful intervention to check the downhill slide the individual is experiencing.

As mentioned earlier, there are some crises which could be considered normal and these generally deal with development. Birth, while considered a physiologic crisis, is less so as medical technology improves, and difficult to evaluate with accuracy as a psychological crisis for the neonate. Adolescence is a transitional state characterized by inconsistencies and lability; while it is traumatic for most, it is probably a crisis only for a minority. Marriage, or the decision not to marry, is another important juncture. It too can cause crisis, but usually not of impossible magnitude, and almost everyone has experienced it and can contribute his or her two-cents-worth of opinion. The crisis is mostly centered around change and challenge in problem-solving techniques ("I like to do it this way" vs. "Well, I don't"). The more acute crises in this developmental concept are those encountered by the aged, particularly in today's society. They are most likely to be referred or brought to a community mental health center, and the frustrations the therapist will encounter in attempting to resolve the older person's crisis will be many: physical problems that complicate almost any situation, poverty or lack of adequate income to properly provide for one's security and well-being, and a myriad of other social, physical and environmental problems which are specific to the old and other disadvantaged people in our society. Whatever these problems are—rejection, loneliness, despair, isolation, vulnerability, or fear—they are usually worse in the large inner city areas.

In Caplan's conception of crisis the idea that a crisis develops from a single event is rejected, except when that event involves death or serious illness.[5] Crises are the result of many smaller unresolved problems or conflicts which are contiguous in time and interrelated in content. This theory is readily validated by the crisis situations old people so frequently present in community mental health practice.

The coincidental crises, referred to at the beginning of this discussion, are the more serious and disruptive situations people must encounter. The crises of war, natural disasters and personal disability are understandably more disruptive and catastrophic than those classified as developmental. Such catastrophic situations are infrequent and difficult to predict. Reactions or problem-solving techniques are critical; indeed, survival may be the outcome of the right decision and death the payoff for a wrong one. When individuals are able to mobilize and cope with such *real* crises they frequently experience an aftershock reaction, and will come to the community mental health center to unburden themselves of the charged situation they have managed to negotiate. Such individuals come to the center to seek reassurance that their decision was a good one, and to validate their ability to cope.

Finally, crisis theory recognizes four stages of crisis development:

Stage 1) Increase in tension as the problem is identified, with attempt at resolution using past problem-solving techniques. With success the crisis is aborted at this point. If not it progresses to

Stage 2) Further increase in tension and anxiety resulting in some preoccupation and ineffectuality. Some attempt to consult others—seek opinions, advice and solutions—is made. This decision may be helpful in finding a new solution, or result in triggering a new problem-solving technique which might work, thus rescuing the individual from

Stage 3) More anxiety and beginning panic as awareness of his situation develops. Increased sense of frustration, anger, guilt, and fear as problem continues unsolved. There may be regression as the individual attempts to salvage something from the situation by lowering criteria for "succeeding"—the "I'd-settle-for" technique. There is intense mobilization of all possible resources, internal and external, that would help in solving the problem. There are four characteristics of the individual's coping at this stage:

a) intensification of the attempt to problem-solve, use of new and drastic methods;

b) redefinition of the problem;

c) regression to a safer, more comfortable level of functioning (also could be defined as sensible retreat or strategic withdrawal);

d) realignment—or "deserting the ship," in which the individual, recognizing defeat and needing to avoid it, shifts gears and moves over to the winning side, if possible.

When these desperate measures are neither possible nor successful then the individual moves to

Stage 4) Where personality changes occur and psychiatric symptoms of personality disorganization, depression, or conversion symptoms appear.

The development and recognition of crisis theory is, in a sense, the third revolution in the history of psychiatry, the first being the 18th century discovery that the mentally ill were neither criminals nor possessed by demons and that jails, chains and religious exhortations would not cure them. The second discovery was Freud's, and the genius of his insights into the emotional topography of the mind is the foundation of modern psychiatry. The third is crisis intervention: a radical attempt to forestall the process of mental decompensation in reaction to profound emotional stress by direct and immediate intervention.

Critics, mostly from the orthodox analytic school, have called crisis intervention emotional first aid. It is that and more. Crisis theory assumes that a deeply disturbed, overwhelmed patient whose emotional resources have been exhausted and who seems headed for a mental hospital can be turned around. It suggests that the immediate relief of symptoms produced by the crisis is more urgent than an investigation into their cause. In effect, it proposes the substitution of emotional "Bandaids" for prolonged therapy (if Bandaids will hold the patient together over an unendurable crisis in his life). Above all, it is a pragmatic approach, and in that respect uniquely suited to community psychiatry. It recognizes that in a crisis situation neither the therapist nor the patient has the "luxury" of time for the patient to come up with his own insights, and that assigning priority to the patient's reaction to his crisis is of more immediate importance than understanding what produced it. It is a flexible, innovative, but reality-oriented approach, and its basic principles are:

1. to avoid hospitalization,

2. to preserve and maintain the individual's function within his family and his community,

3. to assist in problem solving, and, in so doing, encourage emotional growth.

TECHNIQUE OF CRISIS INTERVENTION

Because this text is concerned primarily with the practice of community mental health nursing, and because the authors recognize the increased availability of literature in the field of crisis intervention, the discussion of technique will be succinct and will offer practical guidelines about what to do and how to do it.

The patient's first contact with the therapist may not be at a community mental health center. It may be in his home, or in the emergency ward or outpatient clinic of the general hospital. The contact may have been sought voluntarily, or the patient seen because of a referral. All the nurse knows at this point is that something is wrong, and whatever it is, it can't wait. Crisis may not be mentioned by the patient or the referrant, but the nurse, whose judgment and skill are being sought, should "think crisis," and she should certainly know what to expect and what will be expected of her.

The initial steps in crisis intervention are not dissimilar to what occurs in a noncrisis situation. The similarities, where they do occur, are different in their implicit quality of urgency. An interview will initiate the contact, but it will be characterized by the patient's impatience with questions and high level of anxiety about his situation. He is desperate, something is awfully wrong, and he wants help.

Interviewing in Crisis Situations

To begin with, time is much more of a factor than in a regular psychiatric interview. Because the crisis has temporal parameters, so does the therapeutic process. Therefore, the first interview, while also important in gaining necessary factual data, must convince the patient that help is available, and immediately. The patient states, directly or indirectly, "I am in trouble, I need help." When no one seems to understand or care the patient may act out his desperation by suicide attempt or gesture, aggressive acts towards others, or further decompensation.

When the therapist can impress the patient that help is possible, and indicate competence as a helping person, it is an enormous relief. "Someone hears me, someone understands, someone can help!"

The Presenting Problem

For the most part the symptoms are quite apparent. There is a high level of anxiety, doubt, confusion, and, depending on the stage at which the patient is first seen, there may be symptoms of depersonalization and depression. The patient is generally aware of his symptoms and may have a pretty good idea about what has caused his situation. He will want to give *his* thoughts and feelings about what has gone wrong, and the therapist should encourage him to do so even though the therapist realizes there are other factors which have contributed to the patient's crisis. Wherever the patient is, that is where the treatment should begin. This means the patient should be spared the need to explore the psychodynamic implications of the situation. If the patient wants to talk about his immediate problems and their effect on him and his family (and almost all patients will), then that is where the focus should be. If the therapist insists on placing the focus somewhere else, the patient will probably not return, or worse, may decompensate further.

The History

As indicated, the pressure of time is a demanding reality for both the patient and the therapist, and a more complete and formal psychiatric history may not be possible, nor indeed desirable. However, information is needed and must be obtained in order to evaluate accurately the patient's situation and to formulate the intervention plan. Thus, there should be a shift in historical focus with more emphasis on the individual as part of a social network. This makes sense when we consider our earlier statement that crises are the result of a disturbance in the equilibrium of an individual, and in emotional crisis that disturbance is often in the environment; crisis situations always develop in reaction to something.

It is necessary to understand the patient's social background and to identify and be familiar with his subculture. For the nurse, who has become familiar with the community served by the center, this should be a simple task. Cultural values differ from group to group and from area to area within a society. Consider, for example, the reaction of various subgroups to an illegitimate pregnancy; it would be accepted as unfortunate but not critical in some groups and as a major crisis in others. Similarly, the decision to "drop out" of school would be accepted with equanimity and perhaps expected by certain subgroups, while the same action would cause considerable disruption to another group.*

The patient's history should include, as much as possible, information about the family, its resources, its communication patterns and its alliances (within the family and the community). If the patient cannot supply this information then the therapist must seek it elsewhere from other family members (and the patient should be informed in advance, with the explanation that the nurse will be contacting the family), from other agencies involved in the case, or from any other source which might shed light on the situation without violating the confidentiality

---

*The rapidity with which our cultural values are evolving on all levels and becoming more homogeneous is obvious. Within the past few years the problem of pregnancy out of wedlock and dropping out of school are no longer associated mainly with lower socio-economic groups.

of the patient's contact. In routine situations letters are used for exchange of information, but this is not expedient in crises because of the delay. So one or several phone calls are made. And in a short time the nurse can piece together a fairly accurate picture of the problem, the immediate cause, the family, its probable effect on the patient (negative *or* positive), as well as a picture of the patient. Later, as treatment progresses, the nurse may want to gain entry into the social system of the patient, and if a *gestalt* approach has been utilized the nurse will have better access. This can be called the "no-man-is-an-island" concept of history taking in crisis situations, recognizing that no crisis can be viewed as an event apart from the society in which it occurs.

Other considerations include careful attention to the patient's present and past medical status, including medications, if any, he has or is receiving. It is also significant to learn of similar crises the patient may have experienced in the past, and how they were met.

Finally, the nurse should forego a lengthy intake history and concentrate on establishing rapport with the patient by helping him to unburden himself, thereby reducing some of his anxiety. By the end of the first interview the nurse should have encouraged the patient to focus on his crisis by discussing:

1. What the patient identifies as the crisis;
2. What he thinks the cause is;
3. What he has done to try and solve it;
4. What he hopes can be done to help him solve it.

Therapeutic Considerations

Leverage is an essential ingredient in crisis therapy, and is available to the therapist by reason of the patient's inability to cope effectively with his problems. It is analogous to the leverage an auto mechanic has when an automobile breaks down. Taking the car to a mechanic involves placing trust in his ability to diagnose the problem accurately, recommend a treatment, and estimate the time and cost involved in its repair. The mechanic has leverage in such a situation because:

1. He is the specialist and can, hopefully, repair the auto;
2. The auto is necessary for transportation and without it the inconvenience is enormous;
3. The cutomer *wants* to trust him, and to believe he is capable and honest.

The desire to trust is so strong that the mechanic gains leverage which can be used to set price, delivery date, and other conditions within reason necessary for him to complete his task. So it is in crisis intervention therapy:

1. The patient needs help badly;
2. The consequences of continued crisis are unbearable and too threatening;
3. The patient wants to trust someone, to lean on someone.

These factors give the therapist leverage to set certain ground rules or conditions to which the patient must agree. When an individual experiences real, unresolved crisis he will generally agree to these conditions. Of course it is to be understood that these ground rules are devised to be therapeutic. (They might include instructing the patient to discuss his problems only with the therapist if it is apparent that the patient's compulsion to discuss his situation and seek advice from everyone he meets is alienating both friends and family and adding to his confusion.)

In crisis situations the therapist is direct and supportive when intervening. There should be no hesitation in recommending a plan of action to the patient which he is to follow to relieve tension or symptoms. Such suggestions, of course, must be within reason for the patient to follow through. There must always be sensitivity to and awareness of the patient's life-style, and all treatment efforts must be reality-oriented. Solutions or new approaches worked out in the therapist's office must be adaptable to the patient's environment. For example, it would be nontherapeutic for the nurse therapist to suggest and discuss therapeutic abortion with a married patient who is depressed and suicidal in reaction to her pregnancy without first meeting with the husband to learn his feelings about his wife's crisis, his reactions to such a suggestion, and the religious views of the family.

Crisis therapy is task-oriented towards solving the problem the patient has not yet been able to master. While the nurse will assist the patient by direct and supportive intervention, her responsibility for strengthening the patient's own coping capacity must also be recognized. He must be helped to understand the "why" of his situation and given an opportunity to choose his "way out." Creating options, or at least helping the patient to become aware of options he has never considered, is a good technique. It has a quality of endurance. Long after the crisis which originally brought the patient to the community mental health center is over, this skill, which the patient has learned, will endure. A crisis situation has the potential for increasing an individual's mastery of his environment. If, on first- and second-stage effort the situation falls apart and the patient with it, that does not mean that with skillful intervention he cannot reconstitute and yet master his problem using new and creative measures.

During the first interview the nurse should be considering the probable duration of treatment based on the patient's strengths (or weaknesses), the dimension of the problem, the nurse's own skill and level of competence, the available resources (patient's family, community, other agency) and other factors specific to the crisis. Termination is mentioned early in the therapeutic relationship, and it can be discussed in the context of contract therapy: "OK, Mr. Jones, I agree you have a serious problem and it looks as though there are some things you may be able to do even though you may not have considered them.

I'm sure we can accomplish something together. I'd like to suggest we meet about five or six times and see how much we can do. If we need more time to work this situation out, then the time can be extended."

This statement, or a variation of it, tells the patient several things:

1. You validate his assessment that he has a problem.
2. You indicate your feeling that with some help he can still solve his own problem.
3. You offer yourself as a helping person.
4. You establish a temporal contract with him.
5. You indicate flexibility.
6. You have asserted yourself as the "in-command" person in the dyad—the patient will take his cues from you.
7. You reassure him that he won't always be in the dependent position.

Termination of treatment should be timed so as to reflect the patient's return to a healthier, more competent level of functioning. He has learned something from his experience and, hopefully, has realized emotional growth. He should not be continued in therapy any longer than necessary.

The nurse can use the physically ill patient for an analogy. During the acute phase of an illness regression and dependency are expected and tolerated. The point to remember is that the patient is always in an abnormally dependent state when he seeks professional help in crisis situations. His forced dependency gives the therapist leverage to "get into" his system and to help him extricate himself from it. The time it takes to intervene successfully should be safely minimal. Never should the patient be encouraged either overtly or in any other way to remain a patient when that is no longer necessary. To prolong dependence is to encourage sickness.

In terminating therapy the door should be left open for the patient to return if needed. A good technique is to schedule an appointment 10 to 12 weeks ahead for a "check in" with the expressed option that the patient can cancel if it's not needed. The patient's been there, he's been helped and he terminates knowing he can return.

Curiously, in many community mental health centers, crisis intervention therapy is a task to be avoided. One might suppose that the wisest, most experienced and most skilled therapists would constitute the logical core group for handling crisis situations, and yet this is (from our experience) not the case. By their nature, crisis situations require immediate response. There can be no waiting list, no postponement. The patients can be demanding and their problems always are! For the older and poorer patients whose crises are frequently multiple and unending there is a special euphemism—they are "sticky" cases. So often these patients are "bumped" from agency to agency while attempts are made to deal with the problem, only the attempts are frequently so feeble as to be imperceptible.

Often the problems are a complex mixture of social, medical, and emotional factors, and the earlier referral is made to a community mental health center the better.

But the pattern of concomitant multi-agency involvement along with the usual avoidance of the senior level staff to treat such patients seems to indicate the complications and high degree of active involvement the therapist must encounter in dealing with them. In many community mental health centers it is the younger, more energetic, but less skilled staff who are assigned to these patients. Pehaprs that is as it should be but then theorists and academicians should refrain from cautioning that only the more skilled therapists should be involved in crisis intervention. After all, we know that it is the newest psychiatric resident who is called to see the complicated emergency, just as it is the newest nurse or social worker who is assigned the "sticky" case.

The relevance of this observation is that the new community mental health nurse will frequently be called upon to provide crisis intervention therapy. The authors suggest that for whatever reason this may be the case, it can be a good thing for the nurse, as well as for the patient.

CASE STUDY—
CRISIS INTERVENTION

DISCUSSION

Anxious, frightened, and unable to understand or to cope with her problems, Mary turned to her landlady for advice. She has acknowledged that things are out of control.

Her efforts to problem-solve and to maintain the homeostasis of her intrapsychic functioning have failed. Her anxiety is almost unbearable.

It is essential for the intake secretary to recognize the patient's anxiety. When there is doubt about what the situation calls for, it is better to err in being too cautious.

NARRATIVE

Mary Smith came to the community mental health center on the advice of her landlady. Mary had "suddenly felt like I was going out of my mind." Her landlady had observed a change in Mary's behavior and routine, and although always eager to "lend an ear" to her tenants' problems, she felt unable to counsel Mary. The landlady remembered another tenant who had been helped by the mental health center and so she offered to call and make an appointment. Mary spoke to the intake secretary who recognized the anxiety in her voice and suggested that Mary come to the center immediately. Within an hour of her call Mary was being interviewed by a psychiatric nurse clinician.

As the interview began the nurse was very aware of Mary's anxiety and feeling of hopelessness about her situation. Mary sat with her head down, crying silently, nodding from side to

The nurse recognizes the patient's need to "get herself together" before proceeding with the interview.
These few minutes can be used to estimate the level of anxiety, and to gauge the crisis stage.
The nurse offers quiet support.

By waiting, without pressuring, the nurse begins to establish rapport with the patient who can sense the concern the nurse feels.

The nurse is saying:
"Something is wrong. I will listen to you. I can help you."

The nurse proceeds with the interview utilizing the technique described in Chapter 2, "The Psychiatric Interview." In crisis intervention the questioning is modified and less direct.

The sorting out process, which begins with the patient's history, is necessary for both the nurse and the patient. It assists both in getting a historical perspective and sequence to the situation. The nurse learns about the patient, and that is valuable in planning the course and focus the intervention will take. The patient is helped at the same time, by leaning on the nurse who will take control of the situation until the patient can.

side as though in disbelief of whatever her problem was. For a few minutes Mary was unable to speak and the nurse waited with her, commenting only that "whatever it is, it must be rough." Mary responded with an affirmative nod. The nurse had little information about Mary, only her age, address and the intake worker's note that the situation seemed acute. The landlady had been unable to give much information, except that Mary had remained in her apartment for about three days, missing work but apparently not physically ill. Waiting for Mary to get herself together the nurse noted that she was an attractive young woman, neatly but casually dressed.

As Mary's crying subsided the nurse commented, "You'd probably feel a little better if you could talk about it." Mary nodded and finally said, "I want to, only I'm not even sure what *it* is." "Well, let's see if we can find out. Why don't you begin by telling me a little about yourself. I'll ask a few questions along the way, and we can begin together to get an idea about what's going on." O.K.? As Mary's story unfolded, the nurse began to sort out the information they would need to understand what had happened.

Mary was 21 years old, the middle child and only daughter of parents who had lived in India as missionaries since their marriage. Mary had been born and raised in India. She had been sent at an early age (about eight years) to a church-related boarding school several hundred miles from her home. She found both parents distant and disapproving, and remembered "always feeling guilty" when around them. She recalled wanting a closer relationship with her mother, but felt rejected and was sure she was when plans were made to send her away to school. She had a difficult adjustment at school and was un-

The nurse begins to understand the patient's social and cultural background. The nurse learns that the patient's present problems are related to past experiences.

able to develop close relationships with teachers and other students. She remembered her anger and resentment towards her parents for putting her in such a situation. When she spoke of her anger towards her mother (which was not until the second interview) she began to cry, remembering how "she always just expected me to be a good girl with no problems!" She had not been close to either of her brothers. Mary identified her chief problem as having never been close enough to either parent to discuss her concerns. Her impression of her role as a daughter was simply to be "good" and to do the "right thing." This was expected of her, and in time she learned to expect it of herself. Mary never checked out what "good" meant or what the "right things" were. Of one thing she felt sure: sex was wrong, and *not* good. She had never understood what sex was, and the subject was never discussed in school, at home, or with peers.

On occasional vacations with relatives in the United States Mary felt strange and out of place, yet when it came time to go to college she chose a small midwestern college with religious affiliation. She remembered her years in college as "mostly intellectual." Her interests were religion, music and her studies. She did not date until her senior year when she became involved with a boy who had "committed his life to Christ." He urged her to share his commitment to missionary work. The relationship was platonic. She felt the boy reminded her of her father and consequently she "never really felt comfortable with him. I was always in awe of him just expecting he was right and would know what to do (and not to do)."

The college assumed the surrogate parent role for Mary and a strict code of "proper behavior" provided the structure for her collegiate years. Once, during a summer vacation to Europe where she was on her own, she felt overwhelmed with her "freedom" and became anxious, tense and depressed. She recalled sitting in a youth hostel crying, and feeling "unable to cope with anything." She was taken to a psychiatric hospital and was admitted for three weeks during which time she received a course of electric shock therapy. Mary was badly frightened by that experience, and later, when she felt confused, she rejected psychiatric consultation out of fear that she might be put away again.

After college she took a job as a secretary in a large service-oriented religious organization not affiliated with her parents' church. She liked her "freedom" but felt scared by it. She dated infrequently and tended not to date the same boy more than once or twice because of her fear that "something might happen." She never understood exactly what she feared. She now described herself as "beginning to feel like I did in Europe— having trouble figuring things out." She spoke to her roommate who indicated that Mary needed "more faith in God." Her feelings of confusion and inadequacy continued. She began to miss work. She remembered feeling, "There's no one I can turn to," and she attempted to "keep on coping as best I could." She made two decisions: "to find out about sex," and "to stop going to church." She also stopped writing to her parents who remained in India.

Mary recalled that on one occasion she had observed her roommate taking a bath and "felt strange and excited." She concluded from this experience "I needed to make it with a guy and lose my virginity." She felt that this was necessary to offset her feelings of "being a lesbian."

The nurse identifies this episode in the patient's history as very significant to the present situation. She decides that hospitalization should be avoided, even though the suicidal threat is present. Significant is the repetition of the patient's symptom reaction when faced with "freedom" and her inability to cope wthout the structured guidance of parents or institutional controls.

The nurse prompts Mary to identify what she thinks the crisis is about, what she thinks has caused it, and what she's done to try and solve it.

By now the nurse knows that the patient is aware of the crisis situation and has some general ideas about what has caused it. The inability of the patient to cope is mainly related to her poor judgment and difficulty in making rational decisions.
(Decision—the reluctance, resistance or inability to make it—is characteristic of a crisis. Crises are turning points.

The decisions she has made are incompatible with Mary's expectations of herself.

Dynamic Formula:
Increase in stress and anxiety → bad decisions → exacerbation of earlier and previously latent conflicts → new conflicts → repetition of past unsuccessful coping mechanisms → panic → regression → thoughts of suicide → cry for help.

Things began to happen quickly. The weekend preceding her crisis she agreed to a blind date, intending to "prove to myself that I was not queer." Mary smoked "grass" for the first time and decided to spend the night with the boy. She remembered "feeling insignificant, like I wasn't worth anything. I felt like I was fragmented and somebody else." Coitus was attempted unsuccessfully. Mary panicked and retreated to the bathroom where she spent the night crying "for my mother, for someone. I felt so alone." The following day she returned to her apartment. She felt depressed and "totally inadequate." When suicide seemed "the only answer" Mary spoke with her landlady, who made the referral to the community mental health center.

At the conclusion of the initial interview it was apparent that Mary was in a crisis situation and wanted help. Along with her anxiety and restlessness she clearly wanted to tell about how *she* felt. She frequently punctuated her statements about what had happened with "I don't understand," but it was evident that she had some thoughts about what had precipitated her crisis. The interviewing nurse waited until she had established some rapport with Mary (whose anxiety level decreased as she told her story) before questioning her about her suicidal thoughts.

Nurse: Mary, you indicated earlier that since the weekend you'd thought about suicide . . .

Mary: (Affirmative nod.)

Nurse: Is that a recent idea, have you thought about it before?

Mary: (Crying) Uh-huh—when I was in Europe last summer. I don't think I'd even know how.

Nurse: Have you thought about how you'd do it?

It is essential for the nurse to evaluate the suicide potential of the patient. How would Mary take her life? How well thought out is her plan? What means would she use? The nurse must directly question the patient, without fearing that such questions will precipitate a suicidal gesture. Rather, the patient is often reassured and the situation defused by the therapist's openness about the subject. The nurse must decide what action to take at this juncture. Consultation should be considered and sought, but it is the nurse who must make the first decisions about the course and conditions of therapy for the patient.

Here the nurse wants to know what options exist for Mary over the next 24 hours. She must explore, and if necessary help to create a safe alternative living arrangement for the patient until the situation is less threatening.

The nurse concluded the possibility of a suicidal attempt was present, but the probability that Mary would be successful was not.
(In suicide theory it is the *absence of hope* which characterizes the suicide decision. What makes a situation hopeful or hopeless is different for everyone.)

Mary: Pills, probably.
Nurse: What kind?
Mary: Aspirin, I guess. That's all I've got—unless I used my roommate's diet pills. But she's away. Can aspirin kill you?
Nurse: If you took a whole lot you'd probably get sick, but I doubt that you'd die.
Mary: Well I don't want to die, I guess. I feel so bad! I wish I understood what's going on in my head. Oh, my God!
Nurse: When will your roommate be back?
Mary: Next week.
Nurse: Is there anyone you're close to at work?
Mary: Not really. My supervisor is nice, she's been kind to me. She called to ask if I was sick and I told her I didn't know what I was, I felt confused. She said to call her if I wanted company, or to come stay with her until my roommate came back. I guess I've let her down too.
Nurse: She sounds concerned about you.
Mary: I think she is. She knows my parents are in India. She's the motherly type.

Mary, beginning to relax, feels more hopeful about her situation. Something can be worked out, and someone (the nurse therapist) is able and willing to help. She had no relatives living in the area and it seemed a good idea to encourage her to accept her supervisor's invitation. Contact was made in Mary's presence with her boss who indicated her concern, her good judgment and willingness to assist. Mary began to relax slightly and commented with surprise that "talking seems to help."

The intake interview lasted one and a half hours during which time much of Mary's history was revealed with little direct questioning. The nurse con-

The nurse senses that for this patient psychiatric hospitalization is synonymous with punishment.

Here the nurse:
1. Validates the patient's assessment that a problem does exist.
2. Indicates that with help the patient can still solve her problem.
3. Offers herself as a helping person.
4. Establishes a temporal contract.

In this situation the nurse demonstrates her flexibility. She also acts to increase rapport with the patient, and to establish trust in order to gain leverage. The nurse invites the patient to "lean on me, trust me."

The nurse should expect this call: Mary will "check out" to see if the nurse is "on the level." The patient wants to trust someone, to lean on someone. The nurse has offered herself.

There should be no hesitation in recommending to the patient those actions to be followed to relieve tension or symptoms. The nurse asserts herself as the "in-command" person in the dyad.

sidered hospitalization but ruled it out because of the patient's past hospital experience and the nurse's feeling that the patient could be helped using crisis intervention techniques. The nurse shared her observations of the situation and her concerns with Mary. It was agreed that Mary would be seen on a daily basis "until things are more under your control."

In consultation with the psychiatrist it was decided that medication would be dispensed on a daily basis (Stelazine 2 mg q.i.d.) Under ordinary circumstances Mary would have been advised to contact the on-call psychiatrist, if she had need to, during evening and early morning hours, and the nurse would have informed the psychiatrist of the situation and treatment plan. However, because of the rapport that had been established, the acuteness of the situation and the absence of any family, the nurse decided to give Mary her home telephone number with instructions to call at any hour should she feel the need to talk before the appointment scheduled for the following day.

At the close of the interview Mary indicated her relief in having "a number to call, someone I can trust and talk to." At 5 a.m. Mary called the nurse stating she had elected to stay in her own apartment, but that she was unable to sleep and had again thought of "ending it all because everything is so messed up."

During the conversation Mary indicated she had "so much to tell you, my thoughts keep running together, I can't keep everything straight. Supposing I forget something important before I see you?" She was instructed to make a cup of tea and to write down her thoughts and to bring them with her when she came in for her appointment.

When Mary came in she was less

anxious then she had been the previous day. She offered the nurse several pages of "my thoughts and feelings," and stated "it helped to write everything down."

At this juncture the patient begins to sense that she will not always be in the dependent position. She is reassured that she will eventually regain control.

In a short time, with daily visits, medication, and permission to call her nurse-therapist on a p.r.n. basis, Mary began to gain control of her thoughts and her anxiety decreased. It became apparent during the two-week period of daily visits that Mary had much resentment towards her parents, and that she felt guilty whenever she thought about her anger. She was encouraged to express her hostile feelings, which seemed very reasonable considering her history. The suppression of these feelings was not healthy and increased her feelings of anxiety and guilt. Mary quickly gained insight and was reassured to learn that her hostile feelings *were acceptable.* They did not mean that she hated her parents. Because Mary had minimal understanding of sexual feelings, dynamics, or function she was confused and embarrassed. She felt both insecure and inadequate about her own sexuality. Mary was encouraged to ask questions about sexual function and feelings. She would frequently comment, "I never understood that, I was always too embarrassed to ask. I just thought I was supposed to know those things!"

Crisis therapy is task-oriented towards solving problems the patient has not yet been able to master. Recognizing this the nurse intervenes directly and supportively to strengthen the patient's coping capacity, in this case by exploring with Mary her questions and feelings about sex. The nurse provides Mary with information necessary to end her confusion about sexual matters while increasing *her ability* to make rational decisions in the future.

Within three weeks Mary had returned to work, and was able to decide that "I've grown up so much in these last three weeks I can hardly believe it. I've learned so much, really learned things I never knew about myself and my body. I think I'd like to be in a group (which the nurse had suggested as a follow-up modality) now. I think I am ready for that, I'd like to try."

In terminating the interview, the door should be left open for the patient to return if needed.

At the termination of therapy, Mary asked if she could "drop in and chat

Mary demonstrates that she has regained control of herself by insisting on "my way." Later, she reinforces the therapists' impression that she has regained and strengthened her controls by writing to the nurse-therapist. It is also evident from her note, that Mary has continued her emotional growth. In arranging for Mary to move into group therapy the nurse recognized the need for continued support.

once in awhile," and was assured she could. The nurse suggested an appointment, but Mary insisted, "I'd rather leave things informal if that's O.K. with you." The nurse agreed. Several weeks later, the nurse received a note from Mary indicating "Things are much better for me now. It is hard for me to believe that I was so upset. I really needed your help, and I am so glad you were available. I feel more confident now, and I like the opportunity I have in group therapy to exchange ideas about things that still bother me."

REFERENCES

1. Lindemann, E. "Symptomatology and Management of Acute Grief." Amer. J. Psychiatry, 51, 1944.
2. Rome, H.P. "Crisis Intervention." Medical Insight, 12: 53, 1970.
3. Erikson, E.H. Identity: Youth and Crisis. New York: W.W. Norton and Company, 1968.
4. Caplan, G. Principles of Preventive Psychiatry. New York: Basic Books, 1964.
5. *Ibid.* p. 39.
6. Bellak, L. and Small, L. Emergency Psychotherapy and Brief Psychotherapy. New York: Grune and Stratton, 1965.

5

Psychotherapy

Psychotherapy is that process whereby one human being in a treatment setting consciously attempts to influence another to grow in the direction of maturity. The direction of maturity is towards higher organization and higher integration, towards more capacity for work, social relationships, creativity, responsibility and impulse control, towards increased flexibility and versatility and toward a clearer perception of the self and others in the environment, as well as a clearer perception of one's goals and capabilities. When someone moves in a direction away from maturity he is said to be regressing or decompensating. All varieties of psychotherapy oppose the process of regression in the long run. However, some types allow for a measure of controlled regression during certain periods in the therapeutic process. That part of the mind that has to do with maturity is called the ego. Psychotherapy aims to increase the strength of the ego.

Movement towards maturity normally occurs steadily throughout a person's life, except for occasional regression during times of stress. Under the stress of a common cold, most people experience the desire to go to bed and to be taken care of. This is an example of normal regression with which all are familiar. It usually passes in a few days and progress in the direction of maturity is resumed spontaneously ("I'm tired of being sick, I'm ready to get to work even though this cold is hanging on").

Psychotherapy accelerates the rate of growth of a person but it must be remembered that growth occurs normally without any help. It's just slower, that's all.

The words "in a treatment setting"* in the above definition are necessary to distinguish psychotherapy from other human transactions

---

*A treatment setting, like the setting of a play, is a special situation in which the participants agree to operate within a certain structure to achieve a particular outcome. The therapist, for certain compensation (fee, salary, education, etc.), agrees to spend time while in the setting thinking about and working with the patient to help overcome the problems the patient presents. The therapist further relinquishes the consideration of his own personal needs and problems as being of primary importance while he is in the setting. The patient agrees to work with the therapist on the problems he has been unable to resolve by himself and tries to be as honest and clear in expressing them as he can.

which also frequently attempt to influence growth in a person, such as relationships with parents, friends, and teachers. If all relationships that promote growth are considered as psychotherapy then the word loses any useful meaning to us.

Through the years many techniques and devices have been tried to make psychotherapy work. It is possible to spend a great deal of time studying such techniques as psychoanalysis, hypnotism, psychodrama and transactional analysis, to name a few. However, none of these methods is necessary to call what goes on between people, psychotherapy. All that is needed is a treatment setting and at least two people, one of whom (the therapist) is consciously attempting to influence the other (the patient) to grow.

In almost all psychotherapy situations we find that both the patient and the therapist are growing more mature simultaneously, but usually at different rates (with the patient growing more quickly). If the therapist happens to grow a great deal as the result of his contact with his patients then the work is extra rewarding. The therapist should not, however, undertake to treat someone for the purpose of his own growth. The whole aim of therapy is to help the *patient* grow more quickly.

Most psychotherapy is not done by doctors, as you may have surmised by now. It is done instead by nurses, social workers, psychologists, ministers and mental health workers.

Many nursing intervention techniques are nothing more or less than psychotherapy techniques. Giving reassurance, encouraging, educating, setting an example, appealing to reason, are interventions familiar to every nurse, take place in a treatment setting, and are consciously undertaken to help the patient (to grow).

SCHOOLS OF PSYCHOTHERAPY

A "school of psychotherapy" is generally made up of a theoretical scheme which attempts to explain how the mind works* plus some techniques to be used to influence the mind to grow. These schools are usually named for their founder; some are named after the technique that is used. Examples of the former are (1) Freudian, (2) Jungian, (3) Sullivanian, (4) Adlerian and of the latter (1) psychoanalysis, (2) transactional analysis, (3) psychodrama, (4) behavior modification.

INDIVIDUAL VS. GROUP THERAPY

Individual psychotherapy involves one therapist and one patient. Group psychotherapy has one therapist (the group leader) or two (co-therapists) or none (leaderless groups) with a group of patients. An average size group contains between eight and 14 patients.

---

*We don't know for sure how the mind really does work. There is probably a certain amount of truth in every school of psychotherapy.

Community psychiatric nurses are usually proficient at both individual and group therapy techniques but group methods are used far more frequently, partly because of financial considerations (it's cheaper) and also because they are often far more effective and much quicker. There are various subclasses of group therapy, such as family therapy, confrontation therapy, marital counselling, encounter therapy and psychoanalytically-oriented group therapy. Group therapy is sometimes named therefore according to the school of thought that is followed (psychoanalytic) and sometimes according to some distinguishing feature of the participants (family) and sometimes according to the purpose of the group (affective groups designed to heighten emotional awareness).

LENGTH OF PSYCHOTHERAPY

Psychotherapy may take only one to five sessions of one half to one hour each (as in crisis intervention) or at the other extreme five one-hour sessions per week for eight to ten years (as in prolonged psychoanalysis).

PRINCIPLES OF PSYCHOTHERAPY

How the therapist goes about the work of accelerating the patient's rate of growth toward maturity depends on certain basic assumptions about human development. One of these is that man, and indeed all biologic systems, unless stopped, will grow with considerable vigor until maturity and then increase in complexity until they end. Another is that biologic systems have considerable capacity to repair damage to themselves and regenerate when injured unless something prevents this process from happening. Yet another principle is that growth and regeneration are both orderly and take place in a predetermined sequence that is inherent in the being. No surgeon ever healed a wound. All that he can do is to remove the debris, clean up the edges and approximate them with fastenings while being careful not to introduce infection. The skin then grows together by itself. What the surgeon does is to try to create the conditions under which healing can occur. No gardener ever grew a plant from a seed (although we say that he did). It is inherent in the seed to grow and all the gardener does is to try to provide optimal conditions for the seed to do what it is programmed to do. The seed does the growing.

Personality development towards maturity progresses in very much the same way. Step by step it moves along in an orderly fashion if the conditions are favorable and nothing blocks the way. It takes considerable energy to stop this growth. Also, healing or regeneration after an emotional injury moves along in the same fashion unless considerable effort stops it from happening.

There is one further principle to be considered before going on and that is the problem of stasis or stagnation. In physical medicine any blockage to normal flow causes disease (in addition to whatever problem created the stasis to begin with). If a tumor blocks an air passage, the normally aerated lung beyond the block undergoes pathologic change. If the trachea is occluded then of course asphyxia follows. The same concept holds true for stasis in the circulatory system, the digestive system, the biliary tree, the G.U. system—any place where flow is normal, stasis produces disease. In each case there are at least two problems to be solved. What caused the stasis? What further disease did the stasis itself subsequently produce?

In our emotional lives there is normally considerable flow and, in the same manner, stasis can be produced and cause disease. For example, in a frightening situation we experience freely the emotion of fear and our body is prepared to take some appropriate action to reduce the danger such as overcoming the danger or running away from it. This is the fight/flight reaction to stress. Blockage to this system of flow can occur anywhere along the way. If our perception of the danger is blocked we will not experience the reaction appropriate to handle the situation. If we cannot permit ourselves to fight or flee, then the normal channels of expression of fear are blocked and this energy must be diverted elsewhere. It may, for example, be experienced as anxiety and trembling, as hypertension, as gastric hyperacidity and peptic ulcer. This is seen in school and work situations where fighting and fleeing are not acceptable behaviors and fear often causes extremely unhealthy reactions.

One last principle, using the above examples, is related to time. Consider our emotional growth to be like the growth of a tree. It is simple in the beginning and gets increasingly more complex with time. A given amount of injury to a very young tree can cause widespread distortion to the developing tree, although the tree will tend to assume a normal shape as it gets older. The same amount of injury to an adult tree will effect distortion in only a small area of its branches and be quickly corrected. The earlier in someone's life that trauma is sustained, the greater the amount of his personality that can be affected.

Let us review these principles briefly. Given the right environment people normally grow and mature unless something stops them. The earlier in life that development is stopped, the more far-reaching the results. Healing normally happens after injury unless something gets in the way. Anything that blocks emotional flow causes damage.

With these principles in mind, much that the therapist tries to do becomes immediately clear. In assessing the patient he takes the entire situation into account. How much of the personality is healthy and how much is damaged? When did the injury occur and what caused it? Is the patient's environment capable of supporting optimal growth? Is there a block that can be removed permitting further growth to take place?

THE GOALS OF THERAPY

As can be seen by the foregoing considerations the word "cure" does not apply as it might in an infectious process. What we do look for is that the patient's personal growth and evolution towards maturity be resumed or accelerated as a result of therapy. More than this, we would like him to have a good idea of his own capabilities and liabilities and a sense of what type of environmental supports and nurture he personally needs to sustain optimal growth. Lastly, if his illness is of a chronic relapsing type, as many emotional illnesses are, we want him to be aware of this and to alert him to the earliest signs of recurring decompensation in himself so that as soon as each subsequent episode appears he may seek help to abort it before it can cause any real damage or any significant loss of time.

THE PRACTICE OF PSYCHOTHERAPY

Skills in the practice of psychotherapy take considerable time for the nurse-practitioner to acquire and are learned as much by experience and example as by precept. How one handles herself in this sensitive area is often determined by aptitude and degree of personal maturity as well. These imponderables may or may not be accompanied by a high degree of "interest" in the field.

The community mental health center is an ideal place in which to observe the psychotherapeutic process. Here the nurse has the opportunity to participate in it sufficiently to appraise her interest, and to get an idea as to her aptitude for therapy. It is also an excellent setting for on-the-job training in the art.

Group Therapy

Let us first consider group therapy as it is practiced in an outpatient department of a community mental health center. Groups may be started, run for a certain time and ended with the same participants and no others. This is the more classical situation, requiring the most therapeutic expertise; a certain process and group dynamic develops, matures, is resolved and concludes. It is most suited for more neurotic (rather than psychotic) patients who are fairly well organized and who can wait for the weeks or months until enough participants can be assembled to begin the group, and whose tolerance for anxiety and frustration is such that they can reasonably commit themselves to staying with the group until it decides to dissolve itself, which may take from one to several years. This type of group is rarely offered by a community mental health center.

More frequent is an open-ended, ongoing group where new participants continue to come in and patients stop when they have benefited sufficiently. The composition of the group is constantly changing.

Patients are taken regardless of diagnosis or degree of impairment and excluded only when their behavior is so disruptive that the group cannot function with them there.

The new patient can be started in such a group with very little preparation except to be told it's OK to sit quietly for a few sessions and get the feel of the situation without feeling pressure to reveal any personal problems. Because there are patients already there who have had varying degrees of experience in group therapy, they tend to act as "culture carriers" and transmit to the new patient(s) information about what is considered acceptable behavior and how to use the group to advantage. For example, drunken and drugged members are generally excluded that day because they are not able to participate in a reasonable way. Also, violent and threatening behavior is forbidden because it cannot be handled. Whining and complaining patients are usually tolerated for a few sessions and then told to find some other way of letting their needs be known. In an ongoing group, the therapist usually need say nothing about these "rules." They are handed down by the patients quite effectively. Positive behavior and attitudes are similarly reinforced by the group, and there is a high expectancy of a quick recovery and return to function on the part of each member.

There is a great deal of acceptance of individual life-styles and a person's announced goals to be what he says they are (at least at first). There is also quite complete acceptance of the fact of illness as a *sine qua non* to entrance into the group as well as very strong pressure to move away from the illness. "So you went crazy and lost your job, so did some of us. What are you going to do now?"

Sexual preferences are considered as part of a person's life-style as long as he is responsible and does not cite them as problems. "So you're gay—what's wrong with that?" "So you don't want to be gay, start dating and travelling with straight people. If you run into problems, let us help you with them."

Regarding goals: "You've been telling us for a month that you want to get a job. When are you going to start looking and stop talking?"

All of the above are comments that patients can be expected to make to one another without help or interference from the therapist. They are practical, reality oriented, antiregressive, functionally directed, and part of the group culture. When one patient slips into a particularly non-helpful, prejudiced stance, the rest of the group usually neutralizes him quickly. If they don't, the therapist can ask what the group thinks of his attitude and elicit the necessary support. The therapist does *not* side with one patient against the group or show protectiveness or favoritism except under extremely rare and special circumstances. The therapist trusts that people are basically good and loving and realistic (at least in regard to others' problems) and evidences that trust as an expectation. Rarely will the therapist be disappointed.

Many new therapists are surprised at how many people, with quite diverse problems, are helped by this group atmosphere alone. The words used are often the same that the patient has heard at home. But it is not home! This is not the family. It is an entirely new group of people with no vested interest in the patient except as another human being. He is not being picked at or badgered by people with hidden agenda or anything personal to gain by effecting a change in the patient, and their message is clear: "We don't care who you are or how you got into the corner you're in. The fact is that you are responsible for deciding what you want to be and where you want to go. You are also responsible for getting there. But we will help you."

Some therapists prefer "homogeneous groups," that is, groups within which the members share something in common, such as teenage groups, alcoholic groups, homosexual groups, drug-taking groups, etc. The argument is that these groups bring together people with similar problems and defenses and that they have common needs and share common goals. We have not found this to be true. More often, we find that similar patients share similar blind spots and tend to be too soft and protective of others like themselves. A drug taker can tell an alcoholic "Don't promise us you're not going to drink again—just stop if that's what you think you ought to do and tell us about it later." Another alcoholic would tend to be too permissive or too punitive.

We favor then "heterogeneous groups." These add a texture and variety of experience for everyone that is, after all, the way real life is.

The therapist then is something of an orchestra conductor who brings out the shy ones ("Jane, you know what it's like not to have a mother as a child. Can you share your perceptions of Bill's problem with the group?"), quiets the noisy ones ("Let's hear what some other people have to say, George"), and is the guardian of the group culture when necessary. The therapist is also frequently tested to see if she is for real and if she believes what she says. "Do you really like sex, Miss Jones?" "Didn't you ever try pot?" "Is it true that people become therapists because of their own hangups?" "Isn't abortion murder?" There is no formula to help you handle these pointed and loaded probes. If it is an obvious ploy to avoid discomfort, the group can be steered back to the uncomfortable subject. If it contains another message and the therapist is intuitive and quick enough to read it, then the real message can be verbalized. "Aren't you really asking me how I handle my impulses and whether that would help you handle yours?" or, "I hear you saying that you're still not very happy with yourself. Is that what it is?" The object here is neither to answer nor to avoid a direct question, but to quickly discover what the real question is.

When we can see nothing hidden in the question, we simply answer it. Often what is sought is some comment indicating that we know ourselves, that we are happy being who we are, that we are clearly aware of our strengths and weaknesses and that we are not embarrassed or ashamed of being ourselves. We feel that the patients have a right to know this about us, and often the answer to a question about some detail of our lives will convey this to them.

A nurse who does not hold herself in high regard overall as well as know her foibles should not do psychotherapy. The group experience will quickly demonstrate this.

Communication

In ordinary human communication, information and feelings are sent and received on a multitude of levels from clearly conscious to quite unconscious, through both verbal and nonverbal means. Families and small subcultural groups often develop quite distinctive patterns of communication so that they understand each other easily, but find other groups difficult to comprehend. Families of schizophrenic patients characteristically give conflicting messages simultaneously on the verbal and nonverbal level and this has been cited by some as contributing to the split between affect and ideation that these people show. A so-called schizophrenogenic mother may pronounce words of love to her infant, but not touch the child, or else handle him roughly at the same time. The opposite may also occur where she cuddles him and says "I love you so much I could eat you up," or again "you're so beautiful I think I'll put you in the deep freeze so you'll never change."

Another characteristic type of schizophrenic family communication is strictly verbal and called the "double bind." It's a "damned-if-you-do and damned-if-you-don't situation."

For example, mother communicating with child:

Message I: "Dear, you need my love to live. You couldn't exist without my love. You would die."

Message II: "In order to keep mommy loving you, sweetheart, you have to do what mommy says. You must obey mommy's every wish."

Message III: (Said later, after messages I and II are well remembered and accepted, in an angry mood.) "Drop dead."

If the child does what mother says, he will die. If the child does not do what mother says, he will die. This is a "double bind."

Few people take the time to examine their own forms of communication or those of others. However, it is impossible to progress very far in psychotherapy without a direct look at communication itself—what it does, what it hopes to do—and establish some basic agreement about the meaning of communication in therapy. A start can be made by defining some basic forms of communication and getting agreement on these.

For example: If I say "The sky is blue," I am asserting that I have made an observation about the color of the sky, and that out of my experience and knowledge I have determined that the particular color that the sky is now, is blue. Why I am making such a statement at all must be determined by the context. If we were planning a picnic and you had wondered if it would rain, "The sky is blue" might imply (in addition to the above) that I believed something about a blue sky meaning that there was little likelihood of rain.

Now the sentence "The sky is blue" taken by itself is a *descriptive statement*. To avoid argument, and to make it clear who is doing the describing, I might say "*I see* the sky is blue." Taken alone, no one can find fault or disagree with this statement. It is my description, labeled as such, and beyond dispute. Someone could say, "Well, I see the sky is aquamarine." Now we have two different individual descriptions. I cannot argue with your perception and you cannot argue with mine.

However, when I add the *evaluative statement* directly, or by implication as to what a blue sky *means*, i.e., no rain, then there can be much argument and discussion about this point.

It is important for the therapist to try to use descriptive statements as much as possible and to know clearly the difference between these and evaluative ones. The patient must *do something* with a description: accept it, disregard it, or whatever; but there it is, and it cannot be argued with. If I say that I see you as angry, then you have to deal with this fact about my perception. If I say "anger is stupid," you can get into an argument with me about this evaluation of the meaning of anger, and completely avoid the perception that I may have about your emotion of anger.

It is also very useful to be able to change a patient's evaluative statements into descriptive ones, which serves to "defuse" an emotionally charged comment and make it able to be dealt with. If a patient says "You don't care about me. If you did you would remember my husband's name," the therapist can reply (making the evaluation a description), "You feel that if I remembered your husband's name you would know I cared for you." By describing the patient's feeling instead of reacting to her evaluation, we give the patient the opportunity to examine her communication and decide what she really wants to say. The real communication here might be "I need to know you care about me, but I'm afraid you don't, because nobody does, and this makes me angry. Your not remembering my husband's name is proof that I'm not lovable."

Getting to this real message is important if we are to deal with this woman's self-concept of being unlovable, and the simple device of speaking and hearing in descriptive terms will often accomplish our objective.

Eric Berne (author of *Games People Play*) postulates that we all have the capacity to relate to others in three modes: (1) as a child (because we all were at one time); (2) as a parent (because we all observed our parents at one time); or (3) as an adult. A great deal can be learned about communication by learning this schema and listening closely to others and to ourselves to determine whether the communication is that of a child, parent, or adult. People (including ourselves) often interact with one another according to a certain format which Berne calls a "game." An alcoholic man and his wife, for example, often interact with the husband being the inadequate, helpless victim of his impulses (the child) and the wife being the reasonable, caring, forebearing helper (the parent). Neither can grow in this needy/needed format, neither get the satisfactions of an adult-adult relationship, and both become incredibly resentful. So they switch. The husband becomes the dominant, cruel, powerful one (the parent) and the wife the frightened, helpless victim (the child). Same situation in reverse. Same bad feelings on both sides. The answer? Really quite simple. If only one person is trying to play the game and the other refuses to adopt the assigned role, the game is over. It takes at least two to play.

Helping others to hear and to describe their communications, as well as being clear and adult in our own, takes patience and practice and an unshakable belief that people can and will develop and mature given the appropriate information and a chance.

The "feedback loop" is quite useful to teach a group and can serve to greatly enhance the quality of communication. The rules are simple. To earn the right to speak, each person must first correctly paraphrase the statement made by the previous speaker to that person's satisfaction. No one may even answer a direct question without first paraphrasing the question according to the rules. It goes like this:

Mary: Well, I guess I'll start, and I think this is a silly game and I don't understand how it goes.

John: Mary, you say you think the game silly and you don't understand it yet, right?

Mary: Right.

John: OK. I think it is a good idea because it will probably show us that people generally don't really listen to each other, and how can anyone communicate if they don't listen first. A lot of people in this group seem to have a lot of trouble caring about each other and that's probably as much because they don't listen as anything. My wife has the same problem and I wish she would come in here and try this.

Bill: I understand you to say, John, that your wife doesn't listen and she should be here.

John: That's part of it.

Sue: John, I understand you to say that you like the game and have hopes for it, especially for people who don't listen, like your wife.

John: Yes, that's it.

Sue: Well, I think that it will also show that some people say things so complicated that others have trouble following them.

John: Do you mean like me?

Group: You can't talk until you paraphrase Sue first, John! . . .
        (etc.)

Once the feedback loop has been taught to a group, the therapist or a group member can suggest it be used for a few minutes whenever a problem arises because of either faulty listening or unclear speaking.

Psychodrama

It is frequently helpful in the group setting to create a particular situation for the patient to deal with. In this way certain skills can be learned and practiced, traumatic events relived or troublesome areas identified.

A young man with difficulty in presenting himself to a prospective employer because of anxiety and feelings of low-esteem can often profit greatly from acting out the role of the confident job seeker at the employment office before the supporting and critical group. The other patient (or group leader) playing the role of employer will attempt to portray it as realistically as possible, and the subject will be charged with the task of "selling himself" in an effective way. The play quickly becomes "real" and is of benefit not only to the actors but to the entire group. Who has not felt anxious in applying for a job? What boss has not been unsure of what to ask or what to look for?

Besides applying to everyone in the group, the other clear advantages of the technique are that it can be played over and over until it comes out right. If the setup is not right it can be changed. The male boss can be changed to a female boss; the type of job applied for can be altered; the "script" can be rewritten until the truly difficult-to-handle situation is portrayed, and successfully handled.

How to ask a girl or guy for a date. How to answer a question in the classroom. How to say "no" to the persistent salesperson. How to admit you made a mistake, or lied, or failed, or can't pay the bill. How to react to anger from another person and know what options you have in reacting. How to be sexy. How to be professional and not sexy. How to gracefully handle someone's come-on.

All of these can be played out in a group setting and everyone can have a turn at being the subject and the actors. Sometimes a group member can act as a "role model" and portray a most effective way of handling a situation which the others can then practice.

In many nursing schools this play-acting is used to advantage to teach ways of handling difficult problems in nursing. If you have had this experience there will be little difficulty in applying it to the life situations of your group therapy patients.

The reliving of traumatic events through psychodrama requires more skill and versatility than the above. The events may be recent, such as a painful divorce or death of a child, or remote such as early life at home with an insane parent or acute sibling rivalry. The area to be explored is defined in the general group discussion. The group leader senses that the subject did not fully experience the appropriate emotions at the time of the traumatic event, or perhaps reacted in some restrictive or self-destructive way. A "play" is then devised and the subject allowed to relive the experience, in the group, all the original feelings. The underlying group norm generally states that: "It's better to get it out than to hold it in"; "*Whatever* happened in the past, you can only really live *now* . . ." (and should dispose of the past so that this can happen); "We (the group) are bound to be more objective and under-standing and loving than any audience you had at the time . . ." (so you will get all the support you need here). This technique can often best be observed through a one-way screen with discussion by an instructor until confidence in using it is developed.

The quiet, reticent patient will often be speechless when "portray-ing" himself but quite verbal and assertive when "portraying" another character. In this way a great deal can be learned about both trouble-some areas as well as the importance of role in daily life.

One especially useful technique with married couples as well as others is role reversal. After a husband and wife have demonstrated one of their typical "fights" for a few minutes they are asked to change roles. He becomes the "wife" and she the "husband," each taking the other's point of view, style and language while the argument continues. When, as occasionally happens, one cannot place himself in the other's shoes in any way, it becomes easy to demonstrate why the fight continues. There is either no understanding or attempt to understand the other's position. When the role-reversal is complete, the fight usually ends in laughter and love.

While the rudiments of psychodrama are relatively easy to learn in a community mental health center setting, the nurse with interest in and flair for this group technique will want to take special training in it at a center for this purpose, such as the Moreno Institute for Psycho-drama in New York.

Contract Therapy

This is goal-directed, time-limited therapy, usually confined to one-to-one (individual) situations or couples. Because of its sharply defined objectives it becomes one of the best modalities for the nurse to practice after some proficiency in group methods has been gained. Examples of situations lending themselves well to contract therapy are those such as the young couple with a financial problem, the unwed pregnant woman, the anxious parents of the college dropout. At the initial interview the decision is made to undertake short-term psychotherapy for the purpose of working on the problem presented, with no attempt whatever to delve into the depths of the patient's personality or to re-organize his life. The patient is told "we will meet once a week (or every other week) for six sessions (or some other reasonable number) and no more. I expect in that period of time you will have had ample opportunity either to solve the problem, or at least to be well on your way to solving it on your own. I will try to help direct your thinking along fruitful paths but you must remember that you will be doing the work, not me. These few sessions will be like check-points along the way but the solution must ultimately be yours for it to really work for you and for it to fit properly into the whole context of your life." This is the contract.

Most people have already begun to deal with their difficulty by the time they make the first appointment, and the opportunity to ventilate (talk freely) to an understanding, sympathetic person is often enough to carry them through the crisis. The belief of the therapist in the patient's own ability to solve his own problem usually places the patient squarely in the adult mode, which is of course the best position to be in for problem solving. The limit on the number of sessions also works against the patient's desire (we all have it) to give up, to be a little kid, and to be taken care of, or its opposite, to adopt the parental role and to lecture the therapist on the difficulties of her job, etc.

The therapist must be careful not to make hasty assumptions about the patient's level of understanding or knowledge about the options available to him, or to underestimate her ability to help. We have often seen people of great sophistication and depth of understanding of human nature (in others) show an abysmal naiveté or be just plain stupid when dealing with themselves. The one area that should always be examined has to do with the patient's feelings about whatever it is he is talking about. It is generally far easier for someone to say what he thinks about such and such than to express how he feels. The unmarried pregnant girl probably knows (but don't count on it) that her options include (1) marriage, (2) abortion, (3) unwed parenthood, (4) adoption (and she may include (5) suicide). She may even *think* that one of them is the best solution. However, if it was really all wrapped up that neatly she wouldn't be sitting across from you in the mental health center. She must allow herself to connect up with her *feelings* about her various options in order for her thinking to have the kind of validity that will allow effective action. She might well be angry or depressed, guilty or ashamed, scared to death, or all of these. Once she has allowed herself to *experience* the feelings she has in therapy, and discovered that you (the therapist) can accept and understand them without judging her or turning her feelings off, or running away from her, then she will be able to accept them herself and begin to deal with them as a part of her reality.

It is surprising how many people answer the question "What are you feeling right now?" with "Well, I was just thinking . . ." When interrupted with a statement such as "I don't want to know what your thoughts are at this point, what do you *feel?*" they reply "Well, I feel I will figure it out."

The therapist may have to list what she knows to be feelings (as opposed to thoughts) or build on noverbal clues. "The reason I asked you was because you appear to be at the point of tears. Are you aware of a sad feeling?" And then when the tears begin, be sure they don't get turned off prematurely—"It's OK to feel sad and cry, if that's what you feel . . . It's OK." Never (and there are only a few "nevers" in therapy) turn off a patient's flow of feeling, or interrupt it with your own thoughts or ask why he is feeling such a thing. The patient is probably discovering the real depth of feeling he has for the first time, and when it has passed there is plenty of time to look at what it means.

Allowing feelings to be experienced full measure is as important in the group situation as in individual therapy but is more difficult for the therapist to handle here. As a nurse, your normal tendencies to "help" and to "do something" have been enhanced by training and practice, and it takes some effort at first to realize that much of psychotherapy involves "not doing anything" or rather, letting the patient do what needs to be done. If the patient needs to experience grief or anger or fear, your job is to accept these feelings and allow their expression—usually silently. That alone is "doing" more than anyone else has probably done for him.

CHANGE

It is a human characteristic that "makes us rather bear those ills we have than fly to others that we know not of." Shakespeare, of course, was speaking of the change from life to death, but it is equally true within the context of life. We tend to embrace the familiar and eschew the unfamiliar to the extent that we often appear more afraid of change than we are of pain.

Frequently patients express their wish to feel better, but seldom do they want change. They want to keep on doing things their own way, only they want things to start coming out right. This is eminently understandable, because when we speak of changing something about our personality it means becoming a different person. This is scary. It is a threat to our very existence. The therapist who cheerfully announces "You'll be a new man, Mr. Jones" may well lose her patient in one sentence. Of course the patient must change, but the speed of the change must be acceptable to the patient, not go according to the therapist's timetable. A picture of the end result is rarely reassuring or helpful (besides being rather impossible to draw). We don't climb a mountain by starting at the peak but rather by heading in the right direction and watching the terrain under our feet.

The gradual change from self-defeating behavior to self-fulfilling behavior, from sick habits to healthy habits, represents a change from low-risk behavior to high-risk behavior, and this can only occur step by step. The results in life of mental illness are predictable. The results in life of mental health are unpredictable.

If you cut a test you flunk it. The result is certain, predictable, without risk. If you take the test, who knows what will happen, no matter how much you study? The result is uncertain, unpredictable, with a certain amount of risk.

When we undertake treatment with someone we are asking him to take a chance, to take the risk, that the uncertain state of vigorous life is superior to the certain predictability of the illness to which he has grown accustomed. We ask people to change from their habits of emotional sickness to new habits of emotional health, but we don't ask them the process. Someone who feels no pain will stay where he is, and this is only natural. The really healthy person, on the other hand, will to do it all at once, and we can understand their resistance and reluctance to do it at all.

There is another aspect of changing a habit which must be considered. A habit is an organized way of doing something that has been repeated enough so that it no longer requires conscious thought. It is a labor-saving device. It is (like tying a shoelace) a behavior that, once conscious, is now unconscious or automatic, so that it can occur without effort. If we want to change habitual behavior we have to return it to our consciousness (which takes effort), or replace it with another behavior (which takes effort) and then repeat it (more effort) until the new habit becomes part of our automatic repertoire. During this process our ability to function smoothly is often lost temporarily and for a while we may look worse than when we had the old habit, which at least worked for us. A high school tennis player may develop a fairly decent serve with a certain grip on the racket which he is in the habit of using. The college coach, however, explains that a different grip will permit far more power and flexibility, so the player becomes conscious of how he holds the racket and tries to adopt the new grip. During a terrible period in between he finds that the old grip is no longer smooth and unconscious and the new grip is not automatic enough to work for him. His serve falls off badly and he must avoid real competition until further practice perfects the new grip and it becomes a part of him.

Patients experience the same disability and temporary disorganization as they abandon old behavioral patterns for new ones and must be encouraged and supported to persist until things come together for them again.

Reluctance to change, fear of change, and disorganization when change is attempted are seen most clearly in that group of destructive habitual behaviors which we call additions. (See Chapter 11, "Drug Addiction and Alcoholism.")

The gradual taking of little risks by the patient is needed all through the course of psychotherapy. As this process goes on and successes are gained, courage is developed and greater and greater emotional risks can be taken and finally delighted in. It is high-risk behavior for a shy boy to ask a girl to go out with him. She might say "No." The certainty is that if he doesn't ask, he will not get a "No." Neither will he get a "Yes." If he takes the chance, and keeps taking the chance, in spite of failures he will sooner or later get the "Yes." A few of these experiences and he may become heartened to ask out a prettier girl, or a really good dancer, or one that other guys really admire. Each step is another risk which needs the courage brought by an earlier victory.

PAIN IN PSYCHOTHERAPY

Some of the discomfort in therapy has already been mentioned. Indeed, discomfort is usually what brings the patient in for help in the first place, it is what keeps things going, and is a necessary element in repeatedly place himself in new and anxiety-provoking (painful) situations for the greater pleasure of mastery over more and more areas of human life.

The nurse must learn to distinguish between the pain that comes from bad mental habits and the pain that comes from growing and efforts to change, and to avoid taking away a patient's pain that is motivating therapy or a sign of growth. Patients frequently request anti-anxiety medication but it is seldom used in the community mental health center.

"Miss Wolf, I don't see why you let me suffer like this. I was nervous when I came to the day hospital, and now with all that screaming and yelling and foul language in the groups I'm shaking like a leaf—look" (holds out hands, fingers spread, demonstrating both gross and fine tremor).

"Julia, I guess you haven't told the group how you feel yet, and I expect you're going to feel more and more rotten until you speak up in there."

"Miss Wolf, you don't understand. My family doctor would never let me get this bad. He always gave me Librium—it's 25 mg—and then I felt fine. I know you have some in the closet. Just give me a couple to get me through the day. I'll talk when I feel better. You can't talk when you're nervous like this. It's OK don't worry, my family doctor ordered them for my nerves. What-do-you-think-I-am-a-junkie-like-those-kids-in-that-group-they-wouldn't-understand-me-anyway-just-give-me-one-Librium-then-if-you're-scared-I'll-take-too-much-you're-a-nurse-not-supposed-to-let-people-suffer-Miss Wolf-don't-walk-away-please listen-to-me-Miss Wolf-come-back-Miss Wolf-have-a-heart-help-me."

"It's time for lunch, Julia. Tell them in the afternoon group how you feel about me, OK? But no medicine unless the doctor thinks you really need it."

This probably already familiar example shows how the patient with emotional pain frequently tries to spread it around, to arouse guilt, to manipulate, coerce and do everything possible to force the other person into doing something for his discomfort. Miss Wolf manages to stay in the adult role, although the patient's child-self compels Miss Wolf most strongly to react as a punitive parent and to smack Julia around, or in lieu of that response to be a protective parent and give her an anti-anxiety agent. Miss Wolf resisted this pressure and handled the situation well.

Patients frequently come to the center at first with a pocket pharmacy to prevent psychic pain. When this is discovered, the group process is generally the most powerful tool to use to get rid of the pills and find out just how much anxiety the patient is really carrying as well as being the means of ultimately reducing the pain in a real way.

Patients frequently medicate each other also, but almost always report it to someone so that it will get back to the group where it can be dealt with.

ASKING FOR CONTROLS

When patients are into an all-out child role, something warns them that they could easily do some silly little-kid thing and get hurt, or hurt someone else, and they "ask" for controls, for limits, for recognition of their danger and protection from it. The experienced nurse can "hear" this request in its faintest form and always responds to it though not always in the terms the patient may desire, or thinks he needs. Verbal requests are easier to understand at first than nonverbal ones, which are frequently turned around before being expressed. We will listen to some verbal ones first.

"Mrs. Peel, do you think it's OK for me to have this many pills at home? I mean somebody might take them." (The patient lives alone.)

"Mr. Goode, can you get me on the inpatient unit for a couple of days? I think I need the rest."

"Maybe I ought to have more medicine over the weekend." (The patient is on Thorazine, 200 mg t.i.d.)

These are all easy-to-hear requests for control, but slightly indirect and hidden. As a mother knows her child intimately and picks up cues that are too faint for someone else to hear, a nurse gets to know her patient better than anyone else on the staff and can hear the requests for control in very indirect and obverse ways such as:

"I think I'll quit my job."

"Maybe I can do without my pills now."

"I'm going to New York for a couple of weeks."

When these seemingly harmless and even healthy statements are made by a particular patient, with a particular history at a certain point in his therapy, they may well be heard by the nurse as the request for control. In such a case the nurse should be closely listened to by the rest of the staff and her concern given careful consideration.

Nonverbal requests for control include slugging another patient, coming in drunk or stoned, not coming in at all. These behaviors are usually discussed at a staff conference (two or three staff members talking at one end of the hall will do) to attempt to give meaning to the behavior if confronting the patient does not make its meaning clear.

Once there is a good likelihood that the patient is asking for control, then the assessment must be made as to how much and what kind of control to offer. This may range from increasing the dose of tranquilizer or having another person go home with the patient overnight, to admission to the inpatient unit with full suicidal precautions. Younger staff members tend to opt for more stringent ("safer") measures than more experienced staff. If the situation is skillfully handled, in most cases the patient can be made responsible for himself and the adult self of the patient enlisted to keep an eye on the child part.

CONCURRENT INDIVIDUAL AND GROUP THERAPY

Concurrent individual and group therapy poses certain special problems unless there is a high degree of patient and staff sophistication. In a high-volume center geared to return the patient to normal functioning as soon as possible it is important that the patient be given a minimum of conflicting messages. Unless all center staff hold the same philosophy of treatment—which is unlikely—or unless they spend much of each day in meetings discussing the patient, the more "therapists" who deal with the patient, the more the patient will receive a variety of advice which will result in either confusion or the opportunity to play one staff person off against the other.

The average patient coming to the center expects *treatment, individually,* by a *doctor.* This is what he has come to expect in other types of illness and what he has heard about psychiatric treatment. He will learn to accept treatment from a nurse or social worker or psychologist (with a certain reluctance) and to go along with group therapy (with even greater reluctance). Until he has learned how to use this type of help, however, individual therapy seems better to him, more private, more personal and more effective. Besides, he knows from experience that it's usually easier to explain things to one person, especially of an intimate nature, and of course it's easier to involve only one other person in game behavior. When only group therapy is offered the new patient frequently tries to corner the group leader or some other staff person in order to get a little personal attention.

"Listen, I didn't want to mention it during the group meeting but . . ."

"Do you really think I need to be here?"

"I had this prostrate operation last spring."

"I can't talk to my wife like they said—she's an alcoholic."

"I just got out of prison."

"I have this problem with masturbation."

The best reply is generally "I'm glad you mentioned it. I'm sure it *is* OK to bring it up in group, however, and I think you should."

Adding, perhaps, "Other people have very similar problems and it would be very helpful to the group as well as to you to act as a role model and have the courage to talk about this sort of personal thing."

And "You know, everybody basically really has the same kind of problems. Yours seem unique and embarrassing but you'll see how many others are in the same boat once you start talking about them—and you can help each other."

Many mental health centers do not offer concurrent individual and group therapy as a matter of philosophy. They believe that effective treatment will be hampered by the patient playing one therapist against another. Occasionally however, a patient at a community mental health center arranges individual therapy elsewhere. A decision must then be made. He is told to make a choice between his two therapies, but that he cannot be permitted to continue both at once. Unless this approach is taken the patient will almost invariably announce in group some day he doesn't have to discuss such and such "Because I'm talking to my private therapist about that." This is decidedly not the way to win friends and influence people in group therapy.

Private hospitals and some centers do combine both modalities, but in our experience they spend nearly as much time conferring about the patient as they do treating him.

MEDICATION AND PSYCHOTHERAPY

Mental health center treatment for depression and psychosis is primarily medical.* Psychological methods are also frequently employed to support the patient and to help organize his life along more realistic and gratifying lines. Rarely is there a serious conflict between medication and psychotherapy. However, the nurse doing therapy of any nature with patients who are receiving psychotropic medication must remain aware of the effects which may be due to the drug, as compared to changes which may occur in the patient during therapy itself.

Drugs are often talked about by patients and, unless carefully handled, the subject can occupy an entire therapy session.

"I want the group to help me with a problem."

"Yes, Nancy?"

"How come I have to take Stelazine and Tom is crazier than I am and doesn't take anything?"

The nurse has two options here: to see if Tom has some kind of normal response to Nancy's accusation, ignoring the content of the rest of the statement, or else to remind Nancy that medication decisions are made by the doctor. A third alternative would be to try to find out what Nancy is *really* talking about before going any further. These decisions will rest on an appraisal of what sort of shape Tom is in and some knowledge of how Nancy has been recently. There is no absolute right or wrong at such a juncture, but rather a judgment as to which path is likely to be the most productive.

Charles: "Harry, how come you're shaking, are you scared of something?"

Harry: "I dunno."

Nurse: "Yes, Harry, I was wondering too. What are you feeling?"

Harry: "Nothin'."

---

*There are some institutes in America and Europe which advocate purely psychological treatment for these disorders. These measures, however, are neither economical nor suited to the volume of patients that mental health centers must handle.

Agnes: "I bet he's not taking his shaky pills."*
Harry: "You mean them little white ones?"
Nurse: "Are you taking them?"
Harry: "Hell no, they make me sleepy and give me indi-
        gestion."

The chances are that Harry is showing the motor restlessness secondary to phenothiazine administration. The antiparkinsonian drugs do
not cause drowsiness and indigestion and the matter seems best left to
the physician to review, and he should be informed of the patient's
reaction to skipping his medication.

What to discuss about drugs in therapy is a decision which the
nurse must constantly make. Medication that has such a profound effect
on a patient's being is often a source of worry and concern, can be a
focus of delusional thinking, can be seen as the source of great help or
great harm. The patient's *attitudes* about medication are always fair
subject for discussion in group, however. What shouldn't be talked about
are dosages, choice of drug and so forth that are medical matters and
nothing that the group can "decide," or deal with.

How a particular person relates to drugs is usually an indication of
how he relates to other elements in his life, and the skillful therapist
will move from a pill discussion to the larger area of the patient's life
with ease.

The fearful, distrustful, paranoid patient can be expected to view
the doctor and his medicine with suspicion, to adjust his own dosage
(downward) and to know the names and doses of most of the other
patients' medications. The passive, dependent person will often cling to
his medication, as he does to people, and want more and more. The
depressed patient will sometimes forget his medicine, lose it or occasionally take it all at once. The obsessional, rigid person will take it
exactly as prescribed and want to know the precise time each dose
should be taken. Drug behavior seen in this way, like any other behavior,
can be dealt with as a manifestation of a life style or part of the current
symptomatology.

Drug reactions and side effects are often first recognized by the
nurse in the therapy session and are of great value to the physician.
When 30 to 60 patients are medicated by one doctor in a day hospital
setting, where traditional hospital charts are not kept, it is often left to
the nurse to devise a workable information system to advise the doctor
accurately and quickly. Unlike most other (medical) treatment facilities
with which the nurse is familiar, the community mental health center
staff has few medically trained workers, the doctors are often there only
part time, and the nurse is in a unique position of great medical responsibility. Social workers and psychologists aren't expected to know what
anticholinergic effects are, nor should they be. (See Chapter 6, "Psychopharmacology.")

---

*Refers to antiparkinsonian agents that prevent the akasthesia which may occur
with phenothiazine medication. (See Chapter 6, "Psychopharmacology.")

ORGANIZING A LIFE

There are three important things for a convalescing patient to consider in the process of reorganizing a life that has been torn apart by a major mental illness. He must learn about his illness, the likelihood of recurrence, and how to handle it if and when it happens. He must know himself, his strengths and weaknesses, and what *he* wants for himself. He must set priorities, even write them down, and take one step at a time. The patient naturally tends to remember his life at its most organized (girl, school, hobbies, friends) and usually expects to return to full functioning at once. Functioning returns gradually, as it went away, and help is needed in reorganizing this and constructing a stepwise recovery. The steps must be the patient's. Not the parents'. Not the spouse's. (And not the therapist's.) Here are the sounds of a life getting organized:

"I've got to get my life organized. I don't know what I want to do or where I'm headed. I'm not crazy or depressed anymore but I'm not exactly living either. I can't spend the rest of my life making ashtrays in O.T. Maybe I'm scared I'll get sick again. What do you think I should do?"

"Well, I can't honestly say you won't get sick again. This kind of illness sometimes comes back under stress but there are a lot of things you can do about it."

"Like what?"

"Try and remember back to when you first noticed something was wrong—when you started to get sick."

"I stopped studying and spent a lot of time in my room, writing. People bugged me."

"Right! You started to withdraw. To pull away from people and get into yourself. You also got very philosophical and had thoughts about God and the universe and all, remember?"

"Yeah."

"OK, how did you *feel* in those days?"

"Alone and scared."

"Do you think you could tell if those feelings started up again?"

"Uh-huh."

"Right! Getting sick isn't like walking along at night and falling into a hole. You get definite signs that your nervous system is getting overloaded and that things are too difficult to handle. What would you do if that started again?"

"Come back to the center and get started on Stelazine again."

"That's right! And the earlier you catch it, before you really start falling apart and go crazy again, the easier it is to get you healthy. If you get in right away you probably wouldn't need to stop school again or work or whatever you're doing. What feels right for you to get into when you leave here?"

"That's what I don't know. I ought to finish college, but I don't have any bread. I want to get a stereo and a car and an apartment. The room's OK but I can't stay on welfare and I don't want to move back with my parents. I need a girl-friend. I don't know."

"Are you ready to start studying now?"

"No."

"So you won't start college right away."

"I guess not."

"What's the most important thing to you right now?"

"Being normal and having a girl."

"What do you need to do that?"

"A decent place to take a girl and some nice clothes . . . money."

"Could you work for a while?"

"I think so. If I wasn't hassled. Like maybe drive a cab."

"Can you live on that kind of money?"

"On 70 or 80 dollars a week? Not unless I had a room-mate."

"Have you thought about it?"

"Yeah, I've been talking to Bill Thompson. We get along OK. His head's OK now that he's not doing dope. We could live together."

"All right. Check it out. And the job. OK?"

"OK. My old man will be mad if I don't go back to school right away, though."

"Well?"

"Hell, it's my life."

"Yep."

THE ART OF THERAPY

In observing a fine therapist at work, we are struck by the natural-ness of the process and the effortlessness of it all. The therapist does not seem to be playing a role, but easily and comfortably is just being a mature, caring, sensitive person.

Learning to be a good therapist involves learning some "rules of the road," growing toward emotional maturity and being yourself. It is not possible to be equally at ease and equally effective with all kinds of patients. But it is important to know what you are best at and what you can't handle at all. With a little experience "just not liking a patient" should tell you something about both the patient and yourself. These feelings are not to be ignored.

The most sensitive instrument you have for measuring the patient's progress and assessing his feelings is your own self—your response to the patient. As you learn to trust this you will find great joy in having your existence and the patient's move along together during the time you know each other.

There are no therapists without blind spots and hangups. This is OK. There are therapists, however, who are not aware of what their hangups are. This is downright dangerous. In learning the art of therapy there is no substitute for observing the gifted therapist at work. When this rare opportunity presents itself the student should try to ignore the content and technique at first and concentrate on the attitude of the nurse, the feeling tone of the interview, the openness and the involvement, the caring and the innocent questioning. In an initial session, the expert nurse gives as much information as she gets. The patient feels that he has been heard, that what he has to say somehow matters to the nurse, that there is clearly hope (if only a glimmer) that someone knows what's going on even though he doesn't. The nurse's strength, grasp of important details and honest belief in the patient's ability to get better are greatly comforting to the patient and point at once in the direction of health.

The expert has grace, flexibility, style and ease. The amateur or insecure therapist has knowledge, technique, a didactic method, a "therapeutic armamentarium" which drives through the patient's mind like a bristling battleship instead of moving in the eddies of thought like a swan.

If the student is a curious, open, nonjudgmental person, secure enough to be interested in other life styles, honest enough to say "I'm sorry," straight enough to say "I don't understand," young enough (whatever her age) to be surprised, and full enough to give, she can begin to enjoy the art of therapy in her first interview. The student who needs to know all the rules first, and tries to memorize "correct" responses, will most likely not enjoy such encounters with patients.

CREATIVITY AND PSYCHOTHERAPY

There are two aspects of creativity and personality growth. One aspect involves disciplined expression. The other involves undisciplined imagination. Both must be present. Consider their opposites. "Disciplined imagination" is not imagination at all—it is thought. "Undisciplined expression" is chaos. The artist must be able to dream unlimited dreams and to draw finite drawings. The growing person must be able to conceive of limitless possibilities and options and then to choose those that are workable and consistent with the demands of reality. The processes of thinking, choosing and acting are all in the realm of the finite, the orderly, the disciplined. Pure imagination is infinite, without order, undisciplined.

We cannot speak about the content of our pure imagination because the thinking and speaking processes necessarily operate within limits, with rules. In a truly healthy, fully mature person, what happens is that pure imagination goes on continuously, somewhat like the light source in a slide projector. As we place various transparencies in the path of the light, that is, as we employ various schemes of thought and logic and various frames of reference, what we see and what we show to others is the result of the two things working together. Our pure imagination is the light source; our thoughts are the slide transparencies. Thoughts without imagination are dull and dark and can hardly be seen. Pure imagination without thoughts is like white light—bright but without form.

Schizophrenia is called a thinking disorder because imagination comes through without the order and discipline that gives it consistent, workable meaning. Thought is chaotic and wild, not logical. Obsessive compulsive disease is such highly ordered and overdisciplined thinking that the infinite variety and multiple options deriving from pure imagination are not permitted to shine through the dense organization of thought.

It is as if the slide transparencies of the schizophrenic are too faint and ill defined and those of the obsessive compulsive so dark and tightly drawn that little light can shine through (and he is fearful to use more than one or two slides in his collection ever).

The schizophrenic has so much light that he spreads it all around, searching for definition. The obsessive compulsive has so little light that he holds on to the little he has for fear that little bit will go away. Other illnesses contain elements of these two disorders and can be placed on a continuum from excessively disorganized to excessively organized.

Mental illness is a disorder of creativity and growth. Health is an abundance of creativity and growth. The tendency in everyone is to be healthy, balanced, creative and to grow continuously. Both illness and health are the result of a dynamic interaction between hereditary potential and environmental influences.

The psychiatrist can often modify (i.e., enhance or subdue) hereditary potential (chemically coded in each person) with the chemicals he prescribes. As miraculous as are present-day results of this chemical modification, they are as yet gross and crude compared to what is shortly to come. A psychotherapist can modify environmental influences and bring them more into a position and form whereby they can enhance the health and growth of a person.

Before either of these tasks can be accomplished the therapist will, if she is a good one, perceive the total functioning of the human being who is her patient in terms of the patient's creativity and its expression by means of her own creativity and its expression. Besides a few easily learned technical details, the tool of the therapist is her creative intelligence. Without full access to this, patients appear incomprehensibly chaotic or incomprehensibly complicated. With it, understanding is natural and pleasant, and the patient knows he is understood and respected long before he knows why.

When we consider growth and development the slide transparency analogy continues to be helpful. We are born with our own slide projector and the light source is on every moment of our life. Different people have different types of projectors with various options and adjustments and lenses. They all function in approximately the same way. In our early years our task is to learn how our particular projector works, how to focus it and how to insert different transparencies in it. Further, we must begin to construct the various slides that we will be using throughout our lives. It is as if our minds and memories function as a camera, taking pictures of what we see about us. Gradually we acquire a collection of transparencies that have to do with language and communication, its form and structure, words and phrases, subtleties of expression and shades of meaning; with social interaction and rules about relating to other people, what to expect of them, how they relate to us; with mathematical concepts and the use of other symbols; with customs and laws and rules of the road in general; and with many other things.

If all goes well, we delight in the making of our slide collection, and continue doing it throughout our life. We work and rework the very first pictures we took, try them in various combinations, show them to ourselves and our friends for the sheer joy of it.

If all does not go well, we run into various problems. Some slides may jam in our projector and be difficult to remove. Some projectors have trouble accepting more than a few slides at any one time. Some slides that we make may have such limiting and destructive admonitions on them as: "Don't make any more slides," or "Don't let too much light shine through on future slides," or "Making slides is work, not pleasure, and should be done as little as possible."

The therapist who is familiar with these and other projection room problems can often help correct the difficulty so that the show can go on. One of the greatest pitfalls of this sort of work is in the therapist's allowing slides to jam in her own machine. If her own show becomes dull and repetitive, she cannot expect to help others with a similar problem. The healthy, growing therapist has flexibility, variety, artistry and imagination in her work and induces these qualities in her patients.

FURTHER READINGS

Wolberg, Lewis R. (ed.). "Group Therapy: Part I." Psychiatric Annals, 2:3, March 1972.

Wolberg, Lewis R. (ed.). "Group Therapy: Part II." Psychiatric Annals, 2:4, April 1972.

6

Psychopharmacology

GENERAL CONSIDERATIONS

The importance of drug therapy in the treatment of mental illness today cannot be overestimated. Since 1955, when phenothiazines were first introduced, the entire practice of psychiatry has been changed and the course of major mental illnesses been drastically altered because of them. The emptying of state mental hospitals and the success of community-based treatment would not have been possible without modern psychopharmacology. The role of the nurse in this quiet revolution is central and indisputable. It is usually the nurse who first perceives the need for medication in a particular patient, or the need to change the drugs he is receiving. It is the nurse who first recognizes side effects or adverse reactions and calls them to the doctor's attention. It is the nurse who instructs the patient in precautions to observe with certain medications. It is often the nurse who takes the medical history and alerts the doctor to important medical illnesses, family history and tendencies to drug and medication abuse. The private psychiatrist may attend to all of these things himself, but the community psychiatrist learns to rely heavily on his partnership with the nurse and to use her knowledge and skills to compliment his own. The community psychiatrist working together with the nurse in the area of psychopharmacology delivers a safer, more comprehensive service to their patient.

PRIMARY DRUGS

The three groups of drugs used most frequently are the major tranquilizers, antidepressants and antiparkinsonian agents. The major tranquilizers stop psychosis, the antidepressants stop depression and the antiparkinsonian agents stop the extrapyramidal symptoms that develop as a side effect to the major tranquilizers.

Most professionals, if asked to prepare an "emergency kit" with one drug from each category above, wouldn't hesitate to name chlorpromazine (Thorazine), amitriptyline (Elavil) and benztropine mesylate

(Cogentin). With just these three, over 90 percent of all patients with major mental illnesses amenable to drug therapy can be helped.

There are subtle differences, however, in the action of various members of the group of major tranquilizers with regard to whether they are more "alerting" or more "sedating," particular side effects, and the likelihood of their causing a "parkinsonian" effect. The differences in the group of antidepressants have to do with their tendency to cause more or less drowsiness initially. However, the patient's individual reaction, particular situation, and preference almost always casts the deciding vote as to which drug to use.

> Patient: "Last time I got sick they gave me blue ones (trifluoperazine [Stelazine]) and little white ones (one of the antiparkinsonian agents) and they helped a lot."
> Nurse: "Do you remember the dose of the blue ones?"
> Patient: "Yes, they were 5's—three a day."

Note: Stelazine comes in 1, 2, 5 and 10 mg. While the usual starting dose is 2 mg t.i.d., this patient remembers having had 5 mg t.i.d. The degree of his present psychosis and his body weight are judged and considered along with the facts that he is familiar with the drug and its side effects, that he believes that it will help him and that there is no likelihood that he has inflated his former dose to get a "kick" (none of the major tranquilizers are drugs of abuse*). The intention is to get a therapeutic dose to him as quickly as possible and to abort his present psychotic episode.

> Doctor: "OK. We'll give you Stelazine again, 5 mg three times a day. If it knocks you out too much, keep it at two times a day for a few days but tell the nurse that you're doing it."
> Nurse: "Which white ones did you get?"
> Patient: "Artane, I think."

Note: Patients often know the names of their drugs or can identify their picture in the P.D.R. (*Physicians' Desk Reference*).

> Nurse: "Were they round or like footballs?"
> Patient: "Like little white footballs."
> Doctor: "That's 1 mg. Three a day?"
> Patient: "Yes."

Patients remember difficulties with drugs as well. The man who has experienced disturbed sexual functioning on thioridazine (Mellaril) will ask for something else. The person with a tendency to

---

Abuse here refers to habituation and/or addiction. All drugs have been used for suicide, however.

pseudoparkinsonism who had great difficulty in this regard with halo-peridol (Haldol) or fluphenazine (Prolixin) may be apprehensive of this reaction with other drugs.

In certain patients (new and old) the nurse comes to recognize that their reporting on drugs is qualitatively different from the example given above. The patient who objects to any medication that lessens his psychotic manifestations has to be overridden.

If the patient's last medication experience was as an inpatient, the doses he remembers may be out of line for outpatient care. Too much sedation could make travelling dangerous or might result in the patient staying at home in bed. The chlorpromazine (Thorazine) that success-fully aborted a psychotic episode in the winter can surprise the unwarned patient by causing a nasty sunburn in the summer.

Nonetheless, whenever possible, the patient's wishes are honored, and his comments about his drug experiences always listened to. If there is a clear contraindication to the patient's drug or dose choice, or if the nurse/physician feels there is great importance in using a dif-ferent drug, all of the facts are explained to the patient and his full cooperation sought. Exercising traditional "medical authority" with psychotic and suicidal outpatients is rarely helpful when it comes to medication.

Starting a patient on psychotropic drugs *for the first time* requires more caution, and a careful history for drug sensitivities in both the patient and the family. A family history of success with a particular psychotropic drug in a blood relative with a similar disease is considered as presumptive evidence that the present patient may do best with the same medication. For example, we know that amitriptyline (Elavil) is more sedating than imipramine (Tofrānil), and usually a best bet when depression is accompanied by considerable anxiety, agitation or insomnia. However, if two sisters in a family developed agitated depressions within a few years of each other and the first did well on Tofrānil and less well on Elavil, we would tend to consider using Tofrānil in the second sister from the beginning. Both constitutional factors and family suggestability play a role in drug response and information about family drug experience is sought and valued.

Major Tranquilizers (Antipsychotic Agents). See Table 6-1.

These most valuable drugs are divided chemically into four groups: (1) phenothiazines; (2) thioxanthenes; (3) butyrophenones; and (4) rauwolfia alkaloids. Of these the phenothiazines are the largest and most important group.

(1) PHENOTHIAZINES

Most major tranquilizers fall into this group. The oldest and most widely used drug in this category is chlorpromazine (Thorazine). It also has the highest incidence of allergic reactions, affecting the liver, skin and blood, although these can occur with any in the group.

TABLE 6–1: DRUG THERAPY FOR SCHIZOPHRENIA

(Listed in descending order of sedation; activating properties in reverse order)

Drug	Tablet dosage size (mg)	Intensive-treatment dose (mg—t.i.d.)	Maintenance dose (mg—b.i.d. or t.i.d.)
Butaperazine (Repoise)	5, 10, 25	25-60	5-10
Chlorpromazine (Thorazine)	10, 25, 50, 100, 200 (30, 75, 150, 200, 300)*	150-500	50-100
Triflupromazine (Vesprin)	10, 25, 50	50-150	25-50
Thioridazine (Mellaril)	10, 25, 50, 100, 150, 200	200-300	20-60
Mesoridazine (Serentil)	10, 25, 50, 100	50-100	10-25
Chlorprothixene (Taractan)	10, 25, 50, 100	50-100	25-50
Promazine (Sparine)	10, 25, 50, 100, 200	200-600	50-100
Carphenazine (Proketazine)	25, 100	50-100	25-50
Thiopropazate (Dartal)	5, 10	20-30	5-15
Fluphenazine (Permitil, Prolixin)	1, 2.5, 5	2-8	1-4
Perphenazine (Trilafon)	2, 4, 8, 16	4-16	2-8
Prochlorperazine (Compazine)	5, 10, 25 (10, 15, 30, 75)*	50-150	25-50
Trifluoperazine (Stelazine)	1, 2, 5, 10	10-20	1-10
Haloperidol (Haldol)	.5, 1, 2, 5	2-5	1-2
Thiothixene (Navane)	1, 2, 5, 10	10-20	5-10

*Delayed-release form.

(Note: With intensive treatment dosage, an antiparkinsonian drug is frequently needed to counteract akathisia or other forms of restlessness or muscular rigidity.)

Source: Nathan S. Kline, M.D.

Promazine (Sparine) has a cross-sensitivity with chlorpromazine (allergy to one will occur with the other) but switching to other phenothiazines will usually diminish the allergic reaction. The most serious *liver* complication is obstructive jaundice, usually reversible if noticed in time and the offending drug is withdrawn. The *skin* complications include hypersensitivity to sunlight and various skin eruptions and edema. Nurses who handle Thorazine concentrate, in particular, may develop a contact dermatitis, in which case further direct exposure of the chemical to the skin must be avoided. *Blood* dyscrasias are not strictly dose-related, occurring most frequently in white, elderly, debilitated women, the most serious form being agranulocytosis. The onset of this reaction is very rapid and occurs usually in the sixth to eighth week of treatment. Symptoms are sore throat, fever, chills and weakness. Treatment of agranulocytosis should take place in the hospital and if not promptly undertaken there is considerable risk of death. Following recovery, patients should never again be given any phenothiazine, tricyclic drug (see antidepressants) or diphenylmethane derivatives (see minor tranquilizers). The nurse should be keenly aware of this most dangerous of all adverse reactions to psychoactive drugs and act quickly if sore throat or any other symptoms of infection occur, especially in the population at risk (elderly, debilitated, etc.). Of the other phenothiazines, one is of exceptional value in the community mental health setting, and that is fluphenazine enanthate (Prolixin enanthate). Given I.M. every ten days to two weeks in a dose of 0.25 to 2 cc (25 mg/cc) this drug can effectively handle most psychotic symptomatology. It is widely used in outpatients where there is some question as to the patient's reliability regarding the taking of oral medications. Prolixin enanthate has a higher than average incidence of extrapyramidal reactions and usually the patient is instructed to take an antiparkinsonian agent by mouth concurrently as well as warned about the possibility of such reactions. If the reaction is severe, 50 mg of diphenhydramine (Benadryl) or 1-2 mg of benztropine mesylate (Cogentin) can be given I.V.

The other phenothiazines (see Table 6-3) differ somewhat as to dose and severity of adverse reactions, chief among these being drowsiness, hypotension (especially postural), extrapyramidal reactions, appetite and weight increase, depression, atropine-like effects (dry mouth, blurred vision, amenorrhea) and allergic reactions (see chlorpromazine).

(2) THIOXANTHENES

Chlorprothixene (Taractan) and thiothixene (Navane). Navane appears to cause less drowsiness and more extrapyramidal effects than Taractan and also, like Thorazine, may produce lenticular pigmentation. Other side effects are similar to the other major tranquilizers.

(3) BUTYROPHENONES

Haloperidol (Haldol) is similar in effect and side reactions to the other major tranquilizers. It may, however, produce very severe extrapyramidal effects but tends to cause less appetite enhancement and weight gain than the others.

(4) RAUWOLFIA ALKALOIDS

Reserpine (Serpasil). Rarely used today in psychiatry but excellent for schizophrenics who do not respond well to the other major tranquilizers. Reserpine rarely produces allergic reactions but notable side effects include nasal stuffiness, abdominal cramps, diarrhea, nausea, aggravation of peptic ulcer and depression in some patients.

Antidepressants. See Table 6-2.

There are two chemical groups of drugs with marked effect on depressive syndromes. They are the dibenzazepines (the tricyclics) and the monoamine oxidase inhibitors (MAOI). The tricyclics include imipramine (Tofrānil), amitriptyline (Elavil), protriptyline (Vivactil), desipramine (Pertofrane, Norpramin), nortriptyline (Aventyl), and doxepin (Sinequan). The MAOI's are represented by isocarboxazid

TABLE 6–2: DRUG THERAPY FOR DEPRESSION

(Listed in descending order of sedative and antianxiety properties)

Tricyclic and related drugs

Drug	Tablet dosage size (mg)	Intensive-treatment dose (mg-t.i.d.)	Maintenance dose (mg—b.i.d. or t.i.d.)
Doxepin (Sinequan)	10, 25, 50	25-100	25
Amitriptyline (Elavil)	10, 25, 50	25-100	25
Nortriptyline (Aventyl)	10, 25	25-100	25
Imipramine (Tofranil)	10, 25, 50	25-100	25
Desipramine (Pertofrane, Norpramin)	25, 50	25-100	25
Protriptyline (Vivactil)	5, 10	5-20	5-10
Monamine oxidase inhibitors			
Isocarboxazid (Marplan)	10	10-30	10
Phenelzine (Nardil)	15	15-45	15
Tranylcypromine (Parnate)	10	10-30	10

Source: Nathan S. Kline, M.D.

(Marplan), nialamide (Niamid), phenelzine (Nardil), and tranylcypromine (Parnate).

It generally takes one to three weeks for the antidepressant effect to be noticed with any of these drugs, and the patient must usually be encouraged to continue taking his medicine even though there is little improvement at first. Indeed, the patient's psychomotor retardation, often part of the depressive picture, may seem enhanced by the drowsiness that the medication causes at first.

Once the depressive symptomatology is relieved, there is a tendency to discontinue the medication prematurely. However, the patient should ordinarily continue on the antidepressant for three to six months, and then undergo gradual doseage reduction for up to a total of one to one and one-half years.

TRICYCLICS

The side effects of the tricyclics closely resemble those of the phenothiazines, to which they are related, with the exception of extrapyramidal symptoms. Notable is the tendency to aggravate or precipitate narrow angle glaucoma, and before starting tricyclics the patient should be asked if he has this condition, whether he has experienced eye pain, or seen halos around lights. He should be examined for the presence of injected conjunctivae (reddened eyes). The hypotensive effect is the most serious side effect in the elderly and they should be told (as with the phenothiazines) not to stand up too quickly. Tricyclics also tend to produce withdrawal symptoms upon abrupt discontinuation of a dose over 150 mg/day for six to eight weeks. Withdrawal consists of nausea,

TABLE 6-3: COMMON ADVERSE EFFECTS OF

MAJOR TRANQUILIZERS ....

Phenothiazines	Fluphenazine (Prolixin, Permitil) Trifluoperazine (Stelazine) Butaperazine (Repoise) Promazine (Sparine) Triflupromazine (Vesprin) Chlorpromazine (Thorazine) .... Perphenazine (Trilafon) Prochlorperazine (Compazine) Acetophenazine (Tindal) Carphenazine (Proketazine) Thioridazine (Mellaril) ....
Thioxanthenes	Chlorprothixene (Taractan) Thiothixene (Navane)
Butyrophenones	Haloperidol (Haldol) ....
Rauwolfia Alkaloids	Reserpine (Serpasil) ....

ANTIDEPRESSANTS ....

Dibenzazepines (Tricyclics)	Amitriptyline (Elavil) Desipramine (Norpramin, Pertofrane) Doxepin (Sinequan) Imipramine (Tofranil) Nortriptyline (Aventyl) Protriptyline (Vivactil)
Monamine oxidase inhibitors (MAO inhibitors)	Isocarboxazid (Marplan) ⎫ Nialamide (Niamid) ⎬ .... Phenelzine (Nardil) ⎭ Tranulcypromine (Parnate)
Lithium	Lithium carbonate (Eskalith, Lithonate, Lithane) ....

MINOR TRANQUILIZERS

Propanediols	Meprobamate (Equanil, Miltown) ⎫ Tybamate (Solacen, Tybatran) ⎬ .... Chlordiazepoxide (Librium) ⎪
Benzodiazepines	Diazepam (Valium) Oxazepam (Serax)
Diphenylmethane derivative	Hydroxyzine (Atarax, Vistaril) ....

TRANQUILIZERS AND ANTIDEPRESSANTS

..............All major tranquilizers may cause drowsiness, orthostatic, hypotension, extrapyramidal effects, appetite and weight increase, mental depression, dry mouth, blurred vision, amenorrhea.

.............Causes most allergic reactions affecting the liver, skin and blood (see p. 88).

.............May cause more sexual dysfunction in males than other major tranquilizers.

.............May produce very severe extrapyramidal effects (one of the most activating—see Table 6-1) but has less effect on appetite and weight.

.............May produce nasal stuffiness, abdominal cramps, diarrhea, nausea. May aggravate peptic ulcer. Produces mental depression more often than the phenothiazines. Rarely produces allergic reactions.

.............All antidepressant drugs may cause orthostatic hypotension, syncope, dry mouth, nose and throat, urinary retention, constipation, drowsiness, weakness, dizziness, sweating, overstimulation, hypomania, mania, tremors, hyperreflexia, impotence, delayed ejaculation, headache, confusion.

.............Hypertensive crises (See p. 94).

.............Nausea, weakness, hand tremor, gastric discomfort, thirst.

.............May cause drowsiness, lethargy, slurred speech, paradoxical excitement, ataxia, physical dependence, or compulsive use. (Exactly the same adverse effects as with sedatives and hypnotics—general CNS depressants.)

.............May cause drowsiness, dryness of the mouth, involuntary motor activity leading to tremor and convulsions with high doses. Will potentiate other CNS depressants and meperidine (Demerol).

vomiting, abdominal cramps, diarrhea, chills, insomnia and anxiety; it begins in four to five days and lasts three to five days. It is avoided by gradual withdrawal over three to four weeks.

Toxic mental effects of tricyclics are of two types. The first consists of a shift from the original depression to a state of manic-like excitement and the second resembles an organic brain syndrome, especially in the elderly, being anything from a transient defect in recent memory to delirium.

MAOI's

The MAOI's, while quite useful in some patients not affected by the tricyclics, carry with them such potentially serious side effects as to be considered by the authors unacceptable for general usage in a community mental health setting. If a physician insists on using them, the nurse should definitely caution him in cases where the patient's reliability or ability to understand and follow directions is in any way questionable. The dangers are two. (1) *Hypertensive crisis* may occur in patients on MAOI's who eat foods that contain tyramine or dopa. Such foods include aged cheeses, broad beans, beer, yeast products, Chianti wine, pickled herring, chocolate or chicken livers. The symptoms of such a crisis are: sharp elevation in blood pressure, throbbing headache, nausea, vomiting, elevated temperature, sweating, and stiff neck. Chlorpromazine 50 to 100 mg I.M. is often effective in aborting the episode. (2) *Potentiation of other drugs.* The list is long and contains many drugs in common use in medical problems such as CNS depressants (downs), sympathomimetics (ups), ganglion blocking and anticholinergic agents (used in peptic ulcer and other G.I. conditions), antihistamines, opiates, diuretics, chloroquine, hypoglycemic drugs, corticosteroids, antirheumatic compounds, and the tricyclic antidepressants.

SECONDARY DRUGS

Included here are: (1) lithium carbonate (an antimanic agent); (2) the minor tranquilizers (antianxiety agents); and (3) sedatives and hypnotics. While extremely important in selected patients, these drugs have a very limited use in community mental health as compared to the "primary drugs" discussed above.

Lithium Carbonate
(An Antimanic Agent: Eskalith, Lithonate, Lithane)

This drug is the treatment of choice in acute manic episodes which it can terminate within ten days in 90 percent of patients. It is also tried in other forms of cyclic illness whether or not there is a manic phase, with varying success. Because the effective therapeutic dosage is fairly close to the toxic dosage, it is important to monitor the lithium blood level regularly.

600 to 1,800 mg of lithium carbonate per day in divided doses

usually produces a serum lithium level of between 0.6 and 1.5 mEq/L, which is within the therapeutic range and not significantly toxic. Because lithium is excreted at far different rates in various people, a serum determination must be made frequently at the beginning to be sure the 1.5 mEq/L limit is not exceeded. In the presence of febrile illnesses or any situation that causes a loss of fluids (including administration of diuretics), the lithium level must be very closely watched.

Side effects are commonly nausea, occasional vomiting and mild abdominal pain, fatigue and thirst. These gradually subside and later recurrence may signal impending intoxication.

Intoxication generally occurs when serum levels exceed 2 mEq/L and it produces confusion, coarse tremor, muscle twitching and difficult speech. More severe effects include ataxia, muscle twitching, nystagmus, hyperreflexia, stupor and coma. Fatalities are rare.

Lithium should be avoided in pregnant and nursing mothers until its safety in this situation is known.

Minor Tranquilizers (Antianxiety Agents)

These drugs can be divided into three chemical families: (1) propanediols, which include meprobamate (Miltown), and tybamate (Solacen, Tybatran); (2) benzodiazepines, which include chlordiazepoxide (Librium), diazepam (Valium), and oxazepam (Serax); and (3) diphenylmethane derivatives—hydroxyzine (Atarax, Vistaril).

The antianxiety agents have a limited usefulness in the community mental health setting. As mentioned in the Chapter 5, "Psychotherapy," anxiety normally accompanies growth and change and is an important ingredient in providing the motivation for most psychotherapeutic work. Unless anxiety is incapacitating, most patients can tolerate a good bit of it without medication, and find that it diminishes rapidly as their energies are directed towards therapy and growth. Further, pharmaceutical company advertising notwithstanding, these drugs are more similar to the barbiturates and other CNS depressants than not. They have a high potential for habituation and addiction and carry the same danger on withdrawal (convulsions and delirium tremens) as the other CNS depressants. Of the three groups, the benzodiazepines carry the least risk of the above.

As long as we have a society where so many people tend to get "up" on "downs," it seems wise to sharply limit the use of these drugs.

Sedatives and Hypnotics (CNS Depressants)

Chemically these are divided into (1) barbiturates and (2) non-barbiturates. These drugs have a very limited place in community psychiatry, if any at all. They are all frequently misused as "recreational chemicals." They have withdrawal effects (convulsions, etc.) when abruptly stopped, especially when a high dosage was used, and withdrawal from a severe abuse situation should always be carried out in a hospital. When severe sleep disturbances are a problem and cannot be handled by the sedating phenothiazines, either paraldehyde or chloral hydrate are recommended because they carry the least abuse potential. A listing of popular sedatives is given here for completeness, and not as a recommendation for use.

(1) Barbiturates: amobarbital (Amytal), butabarbital (Butisol), pentobarbital (Nembutal), phenobarbital (Eskaphen, Eskabarb, Luminal), secobarbital (Seconal).

(2) Nonbarbiturates: ethchlorvynol (Placidyl), ethinamate (Valmid), glutethimide (Doriden), methyprylon (Noludar), methaqualone (Quaalude), chloral hydrate (Felsules, Rectules, Noctec), paraldehyde.

Antiparkinsonian Agents

Benztropine (Cogentin), biperiden (Akineton), procyclidine (Kemadrin) and trihexyphenidyl (Artane) are used most frequently. If one does not work well enough after a trial, the patient is switched to another. Some physicians use these agents only after dystonic effects appear, while others prefer to start them simultaneously with the major tranquilizer. After accommodation to the tranquilizer (six to eight weeks) the antiparkinsonian dose can usually be lowered or a milder agent used (Cogentin is the most powerful). Some patients remain convinced, however, that the antiparkinsonian is the real tranquilizer and will not be without it. The atropine-like effect of these agents adds to the similar effect of the tranquilizers and causes blurred vision and dry mouth. If the vision is not improved with dosage reduction, dime store reading glasses are recommended (especially for patients who must read), and hard candy for the dry mouth.

The extrapyramidal effects which the antiparkinsonian agents are used to treat can be produced by all the major tranquilizers in large enough doses. These drug-induced effects can be divided into three classes: (1) dystonic effects, which occur the first day of treatment, up to one week; (2) akathisia, which begins during the second week of treatment; and (3) pseudoparkinsonism, which appears after three or four weeks of treatment.

Dystonia is manifested by muscle spasms of the head, neck, lips and tongue and appears as torticollis, retrocollis, opisthotonus, oculogyric crisis, trismus (lock jaw), slurred speech, dysphagia (difficult swallowing) and laryngospasm (which can be life-threatening).

Akathisia, or motor restlessness, is seen as constant pacing and inability to sit down.

Pseudoparkinsonism is characterized by a masked face (immobile) and shuffling gait with pill-rolling movements of hands, coarse tremor, drooling and waxy skin. Also seen are weakness, diminished drive and muscular rigidity.

It may often be impossible to tell except by trial and error whether the akathisia seen is the result of anxiety which would require more phenothiazine or is an extrapyramidal effect which would require less.

Persistent dyskinesia can occur with long-term treatment with some phenothiazines, especially in women, the elderly and those with some brain damage. It is not relieved by antiparkinsonian drugs and may continue after the phenothiazines are withdrawn. It is recognized by rhythmic facial and tongue movements. The problems with this side effect must be weighed against the problems of continuing psychosis in the population at risk.

ADVERSE EFFECTS

It is especially important for the nurse to be familiar with the more common adverse or side effects of the psychotropic chemicals. Many of these have been discussed under the individual drug headings and are presented here in chart form for easy reference (Table 6-3). Some drugs elicit a sympathetic nervous system response (as for fight or flight) and cause a group of symptoms related to this such as tachycardia, high blood pressure, dry mouth, a dry G.I. tract causing constipation, excitement, hypomania and so forth. Others elicit a parasympathetic nervous system response (more vegetative) with a slowed pulse and hypotension, drowsiness, etc. Still others bring forth allergic responses and many cause such primitive nervous system responses as tremors and pseudoparkinsonism.

Also drugs within a certain group (such as the tricyclics) vary, one from another, in the severity of the adverse effects they cause. Finally, the individual patient's response can cause a great difference in both a drug's therapeutic effectiveness and the type and degree of adverse effect seen.

For the most part these adverse effects are little more than bothersome to the patient, are dose-related and diminish when the dose is reduced, and can be handled satisfactorily without discontinuing medication. However, these side effects are the most common reason for patient's reducing or stopping their medication and it falls upon the nurse, more than any other health care worker in a mental health center, to question the patient about these effects, reassure him, suggest measures to reduce the annoyance, and recognize and report the more serious and dangerous adverse reactions.

When there is a clear choice between having a nonpsychotic patient with blurred vision and a dry mouth, or a psychotic patient without these symptoms, almost everyone will opt for the former. Not every choice is as clear and the nurse and psychiatrist must weigh the various choices together, each reminding the other of things that one has forgotten until the best possible solution is found for the particular patient at the particular time.

FURTHER READING

1. Detre, Thomas P., and Jarecki, Henry G. "Psychotropic Agents" *In* Modern Psychiatric Treatment. Philadelphia: J. B. Lippincott, 1971. pp. 528–620.

7

Group Therapy

INTRODUCTION

Group therapy and psychotherapy of all types have been discussed in terms of growth, change and creativity. All that is needed to learn these techniques and to adopt the correct attitude to practice them is discussed in Chapter 5, "Psychotherapy." Let us now consider some of the historic aspects of group therapy and its development to the present time, along with a brief description of the mechanisms seen in a group therapy situation, and a fine example of a case study by Dr. Eric Berne.

DEVELOPMENT OF GROUP THERAPY

Group psychotherapy is the most widely used therapeutic modality in the United States today. As a therapy movement it gained acceptance in the 1930's, and was established by the mid-1940's. The chief advantages of group treatment for emotional problems and mental disorders are its versatility, economy and effectiveness. It is a uniquely American contribution to psychotherapy and typifies the pragmatic American approach to most problems. The discoveries and theoretical concepts of Freud were revolutionary in their day, but they focused primarily on the individual. Very quickly there were challenges to Freud's concepts and psychoanalytic techniques. The challengers were called neo-Freudians. For the most part their focus was on the individual and was geared to the psychoneurotic, not to the psychotic patient.

In America the psychoanalytic movement was of great interest but quite remote from the problems of the majority who sought, or were designated as needing, psychiatric treatment. The social unrest and pressures of the 1930's and 1940's necessitated experimentation with new approaches. Psychoanalytic treatment was in vogue and seen by many as the panacea for neurotic disorders, but it was accessible chiefly to the wealthy, leisure class.* Yet, there was a pervasiveness about

---

*This is not entirely a myth. Many of the first patients treated by psychoanalysis (by Freud or his peers) were rich, famous, noble and royal, as well as neurotic.

Freudian theory; authors popularized it in their novels, teachers were indoctrinated in their child psychology courses, social scientists interpreted behavior using it, and perhaps most ubiquitous of all was its effect on American advertising (e.g., phallic symbols such as automobiles, cigars and guns). The demands for treatment exceeded the limited number of trained professionals. Group psychotherapy seemed a practical solution. Without increasing the number of available trained therapists more persons desiring treatment could be seen. It was only a short time before the intrinsic value of this new modality was acknowledged. As the practice developed, so did its theory and technique. Before long, group therapy was also popular in Europe.* The initial appeal of group therapy was populist: it was accessible to the lower and middle classes and it seemed a more responsive therapy to the patients involved in its process. This remains true today, and accounts in part for the wide use of group psychotherapy in community mental health centers.

As the new treatment gained in popularity everyone seemed to get into the act. Soon various schools of group psychotherapy were identified, ranging from the simply supportive approach (characteristic of alcoholics anonymous) to the basically analytic approach which remained rooted in the psychoanalytic techniques of transference, free association and dream interpretation. It is not possible to conduct traditional psychoanalysis in groups. Most people aren't interested in other's dreams, and free association by a group of four or five people does not enhance communication between the members but only produces chaos. Some therapists cling to what they know best however irrelevant it may be to the situation or the patient. Many studies were initiated to validate the impressions and hypotheses group therapists were describing. A definite pattern of group interaction and process was defined and the study of group dynamics was formulated. Some of the early writers and theorists the student should be familiar with are S. R. Slavson, J. L. Moreno, C. R. Rogers, K. Lewin and S. Freud. Of course there are many others, and their numbers grow yearly as new variations on the group therapy theme are described.

An important development in the practice of group therapy is that many nonpsychiatrists became active in the treatment process. Psychologists, social workers and educators made contributions to group theory. Slavson, whose original contributions to the literature are basic and who continues to practice and comment, was an engineer when he moved into the area of group psychotherapy. Certain names are associated with specific approaches to group therapy, and although the authors suggest an eclectic approach to all psychotherapy it is helpful to be familiar with who did what, and why. The technique of psychodrama discussed in Chapter 5 was developed by Jacob L. Moreno. In psychodrama the therapist is the "director," casting the patients (actors)

---

* Alfred Adler was the first European psychiatrist to use the new approach. Jacob L. Moreno, the psychodramatist, is recognized as the first to refer to the technique as group psychotherapy in 1931.

according to her knowledge of their personalities and her decision about what role would be most helpful to each patient. Psychodrama is useful as a group therapy technique when the therapist wants to gauge the perceptions, awareness and insight a group member has about another or about others in the group. Moreno was interested in how individuals perceive each other, and by developing the role-playing method and integrating it into a group therapy approach he provided therapists with a new technique that could be used to expand a patient's capacity to experience another's expectations, fears and anxieties. As a didactic tool for patients in a therapy group it is valuable because it greatly helps to clarify the distortions that exist in interpersonal relations. The role-playing technique is widely used today by all kinds of political, social, religious and educational training groups.

Another theorist who contributed to group theory was Kurt Lewin, a psychologist. Lewin observed the rise of Nazism in Germany in the early 1930's and his awareness of social problems was converted to astute commentary about social forces, social changes and a leader's effect on groups. He made major contributions to the theory of group dynamics, and his early studies dealt with the structure and functioning of groups, the group "climate" and the impact of leaders on groups. Lewin showed that it is easier to bring about change in individuals in a group setting than in one-to-one therapy. It has been demonstrated that "when an individual is confronted with a majority group opinion that is contrary to his own . . . he will commonly change his opinions to conform with those of the group."[1] Groups exert considerable control on their members to conform. Defiance or nonconformity is punished; compliance is rewarded. The rewards of "playing by the rules" are proportionate to the investment the individual has in membership in the group. This is important for the therapist to understand because in group process the member, or patient, experiences a sense of group feeling which signals to him that he "belongs." When membership in the group is valued, as it usually is, patients will try to adjust their behavior in order to gain greater acceptance and recognition by the group. This is desirable because it assists the patient in changing unwanted behavior which has prompted him to seek treatment in the first place. Symptom relief can be temporary or permanent, and in a well-run therapy group there can be obvious changes in an individual and his behavior towards others.

Group therapy, as it has evolved over the past several decades, has demonstrated its relevance to the needs of the community and, as we indicated earlier, it is the treatment of choice in many community mental health centers. Inpatient, outpatient and partial hospital units all find the group approach both workable and therapeutic. It can be used alone or in special situations together with individual or family therapy sessions.

GROUP MECHANISMS

There are certain mechanisms operating in groups which attract and engage the members in the group process, and which facilitate change and health.[2] These mechanisms are common to all therapy groups.

Group Acceptance

Group members generally have a sense of acceptance, belonging, respect, and comfort in the group. These feelings develop over several meetings, and intensify as the group gains cohesiveness.

Reality Testing

In a group members can check reactions to their behavior, opinions, and feelings (about themselves and others) openly and in a non-threatening atmosphere. Members can give and get feedback from other members.

Universalization

Finding out that others have the same or similar problems is reassuring to group members. It may be the first time the member learns that his problem is not unique, and that he is not different.

Ventilation

Group members have an opportunity in a safe setting to ventilate (express or let out) anger, anxiety, fear, fantasy, guilt or other strong emotional feelings which would otherwise remain repressed. The chance to "get it off my chest" and to "tell it like it is" is an extremely important aspect of group process.

Intellectualization

Through this mechanism group members become more aware of others, begin to understand "what makes people tick," gain insight, and learn to evaluate symptoms in themselves and in others.

Altruism

This term refers to the phenomenon of group members giving support, advice, encouragement and love to one another.

Transference

Here a strong emotional attachment of one member to another, to the therapist, or to the entire group develops.

Interaction

Through interaction with others in the group each member is helped to assert himself and to increase his capacity for interacting with others outside of the group.

CASE STUDY

The following group therapy session is presented to demonstrate the effectiveness of the approach when used in an inpatient setting. It is offered with its original introduction and postgroup discussion which explain the therapist's approach to group therapy.°

This report is based on a group therapy meeting in a closed ward . . . Eric Berne, M.D., . . . conducted the meeting, utilizing the technique of transactional psychotherapy, of which he (was) the leading proponent. An important concept in transactional psychotherapy is that "the child" in a patient may take over the adult "inappropriately or unproductively." When it does, the "complete, well-structured adult . . . needs to be uncovered or activated." This concept was employed in the first part of the meeting, a therapy session with ten younger inpatients. An equal number of older inpatients functioned as observers during the meeting and were then asked by Dr. Berne to comment on what happened. He then asked the staff for their opinions. (The two groups alternate, the younger patients functioning as "patients" one week and as "observers" the next week, with the older patients alternating likewise.) The "inpatients" formed an inner circle with their chairs, the patient-observers sat in an outer circle.

Therapy Session of Inpatients

Pearl: Dr. Berne, shouldn't we all be introduced before we start?

Dr. Berne: Not particularly.

Pearl: This is our dayroom. When strangers come—

Sam: We haven't time to waste.

Tom: Dumb ass! Every time Pearl says something, I know we're going off on a tangent.

Sam: Dr. Berne, why does a man have to stay in a hospital for eight weeks when he wants out?

Dr. Berne: What does he have to do to get in?

Sam: I just worked a little harder than the average.

Dr. Berne: What did you do that caused people to say you had to go to the hospital?

°Reprinted with permission from the Roche Report, "Frontiers of Hospital Psychiatry, 7 (10): May 1970, pp. 5-8.

Sam:	They got uncomfortable with the way I was acting. I thought I was acting pretty good.
Dr. Berne:	How were you acting?
Sam:	Working fast all day long. That's all.
Dr. Berne:	Sounds all right to me. Why would someone put you in the hospital because you were working fast?
Sam:	I've asked that question for three weeks.
Dr. Berne:	What did you do to get in the hospital?
Sam:	I asked for help. I said I needed a vacation in some far-off place. The doctor immediately said I had to go to the hospital.
Dr. Berne:	What did you do to get in the hospital?
Sam:	I was working 18 hours a day, sleeping four—having a grand time.
Dr. Berne:	The reason you're here is because you don't answer questions. I still don't know why you're in the hospital.
Sam:	I was losing control.
Dr. Berne:	What did you do when you lost control?
Sam:	Worked like two men.
Dr. Berne:	Okay, that's why you're in the hospital.
Sam:	How can they expect you to gain control when 18 people are telling you what to do?
Dr. Berne:	I don't know.
Sam:	I feel worse in the hospital than I did on the outside.
Emilio:	Brother, find a way of talking to the doctor who signs the paper saying you're cured.
Ruth:	You don't want to change, Sam.
Sam:	'Course not!
David:	Dr. Berne, I've just been here a few days. I need a little help. I can't get along with people. I always have to have one guy I don't like, and when I quit not liking him, there's someone else I don't like. In the short time I've been here, I'm already mad at half the guys. I've been working on myself for 10 years and not getting anywhere.
Dr. Berne:	What do you ask of life?
David:	I'd like to be comfortable working with people— have a steady job so I could accomplish things, like buying a house. I can't look forward to anything now because I don't know from one day to the next if I'm going to blow up.
Pearl:	You told me you get along with your mother and you work well with women.
Dr. Berne:	How come you only want a little help?
David:	I don't want a little help; I want help.

Dr. Berne:	You said "a little help."
David:	I've gone to a psychiatrist, and I've been in a state hospital twice. I found out that nobody can help you a whole lot. They give you a little bit, and you've got to do the rest yourself.
Dr. Berne:	You're not really thinking. All you're doing is saying, "Oh, the tragedy of it." How come you only want a little help? You're really saying you don't want to get better.
Pearl:	You told me last week the child part of you didn't want to get better and the adult part of you did. Don't forget a part of your personality is the free child. You need to learn to let the free child express himself.
Maria:	What do you mean by free child?
Pearl:	Dr. Berne explained it in his book. In every adult there's a free child who wants to run on the beach, make love, enjoy things, be happy.
Dr. Berne:	Okay, Pearl. I'd like to talk about a few things with David. What did your parents tell you about life?
David:	I don't know. My mother and father were divorced when I was six, and she married again. I never talked to my stepfather. He's so stern.
Dr. Berne:	What did your mother tell you about life when you were young?
David:	I don't know. She wanted me to be a lawyer or something. I stayed with her parents for a while after the divorce. My grandfather was a very grouchy man.
Dr. Berne:	What did he say to you when he was grouchy?
David:	"Goddamn you, kid, I'll take a razor strap to you if you don't do those dishes." He scared me. My stepfather scared me too.
Dr. Berne:	What did your stepfather say to you?
David:	Him! All he tried to do was make money.
Dr. Berne:	What did he say to you?
David:	"If you don't shut up, I'll knock your head off." He gave me an inferiority complex. I can't walk down the street without fear. I haven't any confidence.
Dr. Berne:	Okay. What did your grandfather say?
David:	He said he'd beat the hell out of me, that I'd never amount to anything.
Dr. Berne:	How did he say it?
David:	I think he said "That kid. I don't like him."
Dr. Berne:	How about answering my question? What did your grandfather say to you?

David:	He said he'd knock the hell out of me if I didn't straighten up and do the dishes.
Dr. Berne:	And what did your stepfather say?
David:	"I'll knock your head off."
Dr. Berne:	What did your mother say?
David:	She never said anything. She went along with my stepfather. But when it came to doing anything, I had to ask her.
Dr. Berne:	What did she say when you asked her?
David:	She wouldn't let me go. Like going in a boat. She was afraid I'd drown. She was a worrier. I sometimes think I picked up worrying from her.
Ruth:	Do you lack confidence in yourself?
Dr. Berne:	Why did you ask David if he lacked confidence in himself?
Ruth:	Because I lack it myself.
Dr. Berne:	He already said he lacked confidence; so why did you ask him, and why do you want to know whether he lacks it or not?
Ruth:	Because I like support from other people.
Dr. Berne:	Why is it supportive when he says he lacks confidence?
Ruth:	It's good to know someone else lacks confidence. It makes me feel better.
Pearl:	David, does it make you feel more comfortable?
Dr. Berne:	Hold it, Pearl. I want to get back to David. What you've really been saying, David, is that you don't want to get better. If you can find a few people who feel like you do, you won't have to get better.
Ruth:	That doesn't make sense to me.
Dr. Berne:	Why? You said it makes you feel better; if someone else lacks confidence, it makes you more comfortable.
Ruth:	I follow you.
Dr. Berne (to Tom):	Which of your parents doesn't like you?
Tom:	My father. He thinks I'm stupid. He calls me a dumb-ass kid.
Dr. Berne:	Okay, so why are you like your father?
Tom:	I'm not like him!
Dr. Berne:	When we first started this session, you called Pearl a dumb ass, and you've muttered it each time she said something.
Tom:	She is a dumb ass!
Dr. Berne:	I don't know about that. (Laughter) The point is you say the same thing to her that your father says to you.

Tom: It's grown into me, I guess.

Dr. Berne: Is that the way you want it?

Tom: No.

Dr. Berne: What are you going to do about it?

Tom: Have patience with people.

Dr. Berne: Is that what your mother says? Have patience with people?

Tom: Yeah.

Dr. Berne: Have you any thoughts of your own—thoughts that aren't your mother's or father's?

Tom: Sure, I do!

Dr. Berne: Let's hear one. When you talk to Pearl, it's your father. When you say, "Have patience," it's your mother. Now what do you say?

Tom: Whew! It's not one way or another. You got to find a happy medium.

Dr. Berne: That's your mother too. Can you say something of your own?

Tom: I'm not going to say Pearl is stupid anymore. I'll just keep it all inside of me.

Ruth: You use the same technique with us. When you don't want to be bothered, you clam up. That's because you're trying to fight society and its institutions.

Dr. Berne: I don't blame you for fighting institutions, because you have two institutions in your head telling you what to do all the time. I still haven't heard you say something that you think independently of your father or mother.

Tom: I want to get out of this place!

Dr. Berne: Okay. That's a beginning. Can you think of something else?

Tom: I want to be liked by everyone.

Maria: I can understand that you want to be liked by people. I do too. But sometimes we go at it the wrong way. To tell girls you'll get a knife and go after them, that's sadistic.

Tom: You think I'd chicken out? Do you know how many birds I've killed? I used to stick birds in the washing machine and then put it on spin.

Maria: I don't want to talk to you. You're a maniac. You're sick. It's good you're in the hospital. I want out, but I'm glad you're in. (Laughter)

Emilio: I have a gun, and sometimes I do things that are illegal. The other day I shot blackbirds. You know what I made? Spaghetti sauce.

Sam: What's your problem, Emilio?

Emilio:	God knows.
Pearl:	You're not coming on straight. They wouldn't let you go into the kitchen because you were on suicide precaution.
David:	What put you in the hospital?
Emilio:	I came to be circumcised. It's a nuisance to have to wash that thing every day. What if you don't have any water?
Sam:	You told me you couldn't sleep.
Emilio:	Because there's a Why? in my head. Why doesn't Pope Paul recognize us properly? I have kids. And maybe, when they grow up, they'll get married and divorced. They say in heaven you sit in a circle, and I want my kids to sit in the circle with me.
Dr. Berne:	What crazy thing did you do to get in the hospital?
Emilio:	I went to the emergency room.
Dr. Berne:	To get a circumcision?
Emilio:	Yes. And the doctor asked me why I wanted to do it and I told him—
Dr. Berne:	Okay. It would take a lot of time to give all the details. Let's hear from people who haven't said anything. (Turning to Mary) Mary, what about you? How did you get here?
Mary:	I didn't do anything. I just don't think right.
Dr. Berne:	What were you thinking?
Mary:	I didn't want to go places.
Pearl:	There is something wrong with you, Mary. You went to college and trained to be a teacher, and then you were afraid to go out in the world. You stayed at home to be protected by your mother and you worked in your father's office.
Dr. Berne:	You don't go to the hospital because you work for your father.
Mary:	I told him I couldn't take it anymore. I blew. I was afraid I'd kill myself.
Dr. Berne:	And anyone else?
Mary:	Only my parents. I took a room by myself, but it was too lonely; so I went back home, and I—I—I (becomes incoherent).
Dr. Berne:	Okay. (To Bob) You haven't said anything.
Bob:	I set my room on fire.
Dr. Berne:	Why did you do that?
Bob:	I thought the world was coming to an end, and I might as well start it off.

Dr. Berne: Why are you in a hurry to end the world? Why can't you let it happen? Why do you have to help?

Bob: I don't know.

Dr. Berne: Is there someone you want to die?

Bob: I guess myself.

Dr. Berne: There must be somebody else you want to knock off if you're set on ending the whole world.

Pearl: He smokes marijuana.

Dr. Berne: Do you know why you wanted to end the world?

Bob: I just wanted everything to be over.

Dr. Berne: What did your parents say to you when you were young? Do you remember anything they said?

Bob: No.

Dr. Berne: Do you still want to get it over with?

Bob: No.

Dr. Berne: Okay, I guess that's all we have time for today. Will the groups change places now? (The younger patients move to the outer circle. The older patients take the chairs in the inner circle.)

Discussion With Older Patients

Dr. Berne: If you can only talk about your own troubles, you should do it here. You were supposed to be listening to what went on. You may have something to say about the younger patients.

Male Patient
Observer: I was in a group with Pearl at one time. She just doesn't want to be an adult. Emilio is terribly hung up on religion.

Dr. Berne: We're here to help people get better. What do you think we ought to do to help Pearl?

Male Patient: Staff and patients should try to make Pearl realize that she's an adult. Otherwise she'll be in institutions the rest of her life.

Dr. Berne: What about Emilio? How would you help him?

Male Patient: I have no idea. (Dr. Berne asks the older patients for ideas on helping the younger patients. Except for one woman the others have no comments.)

Female Patient: Pearl should stop having babies. Every time she has one she lands in here. She's had her share, and so have I. We both need to get some joy out of life.

Dr. Berne: What do you think about Mary?

Female Patient: I'm fond of her. Maria has beautiful children, and they need a father. I told her so. I told her she should marry a man with money. And that boy Tom! Why, he ought to go to school and obey his parents. I obeyed mine. Till I was 18 I didn't open my mouth.

Dr. Berne: Okay. Any others? If not, then let's hear what the staff has to say.

Discussion With Staff

Nurse 1: Pearl is really better now. But she doesn't listen. She only picks up a word or two so she can interrupt. She tried to cut you off when you were talking to patients.

Dr. Berne: That's one of the jobs of a group therapist—to keep patients from cutting others off.

Nurse 2: Most patients were angry, and they went at each other in an angry way, but they rarely said why they were angry. It would be better if they could come out straight and say what it is about a person that's making them angry. Take Emilio. He keeps interrupting, but he doesn't say what is angering him or why.

Dr. Berne: If he did, who would it help? The patient or Emilio?

Nurse 2: Both. Emilio could hear how he was coming along in the group, and the patient would be helped too.

Nurse 3: I was disappointed that those in the outer circle who were really listening didn't feel comfortable enough to say how they felt about what happened.

Nurse 4: I got the feeling that Pearl wanted to become the leader of the group.

Nurse 5: This is the first time I heard David speak about his father or grandfather. It was as if he was making a bridge to his difficulties.

Nurse 6: I was interested in your observation that Ruth can't come out and say she feels this way until someone says they feel this way.

Second-Year Resident: Some patients cannot stand to see others get well. Pearl tried to sabotage anything going on. Ruth was more subtle about it. Emilio would come out with a lot of trash anytime you were making progress with a patient.

Dr. Berne: Any other staff people? No? Then let me summarize a few things in this very complicated
deal. The first thing that interested me was that
when everybody was sitting close to each other
in a circle they talked more to each other than
when they sat at a table at other sessions. I think
the idea of having other patients listen is rather
good. I can't say the listeners contributed very
much, but I think if we did this regularly they
would start thinking. (Note: This was strongly
borne out by later experiences.)

As far as the inner group is concerned: Tom,
who likes to cut and kill birds, only repeats
what his mother and father say. There must be
an adult in Tom. Try to get to the adult. You
could wander off with him, trying to find out
why he wants to shoot birds, but it would be
a waste of time. It would take years. So instead
of analyzing, try to get to the adult in Tom. Then
he might start to get better.

The same thing applies to Ruth. I was interested in that maneuver with David. When
he said he felt inferior, she asked him if he ever
felt inferior. One thing she was after was to be
comfortable while feeling inferior. But there's
something else there I don't understand. Whatever it is, it's very pervasive. She's playing some
game, and she's doing it 90% of the time.

I think Pearl's child is out so much that you
have to make the child feel better before she
can be an adult. That's the way to approach her.

About Sam, who wants out. Don't bother
him. Let him rest for one or two weeks. Some
people come to the hospital for a vacation. They
will do all kinds of things to get in a hospital.
They probably want a vacation, and they are
entitled to one.

As for David, he probably has said all the
things he said here when he was in a state hospital. He probably was told he was a masochist,
had homosexual tendencies and so forth, and it
didn't do any good. All the psychodynamic
formulations are irrelevant in his case. The key
thing he said here was that he wanted a little
help. When he says he wants a lot of help, you'll
be in a much better position to help him. That
would mean he really wants to get well.

> That's about all we have time for. Next week we'll reverse the circles and see what happens.

This example is useful because it includes sufficient dialogue for the reader to get the *feel* of the group process, and to check out questions about the therapist's technique and his interpretation of the group interaction. (The reader is referred to Chapter 5 "Psychotherapy," for additional discussion and description of group therapy.)

REFERENCES

1. Rosenbaum, M. and Berger, M. (eds.). Group Psychotherapy and Group Function. New York: Basic Books, 1963. p. 16.
2. Corsini, R. J. and Rosenberg, B. "Mechanisms of Group Psychotherapy: Processes and Dynamics." *In* Rosenbaum, M. and Berger, M. (eds.). Group Psychotherapy and Group Function. New York: Basic Books, 1963. pp. 342-343.

FURTHER READING

Berne, E. Principles of Group Treatment. New York: Oxford University Press, 1966.

National Training Laboratories, National Education Association, Manual on Group Development.

Shaskan, Donald A. "Group Psychotherapy: Present Trends in Management of the More Severe Emotional Problems." Psychiatric Annals, 2:4, April 1972.

Watzlawick, P., Beavin, J. and Jackson, D. Pragmatics of Human Communication. New York: W. W. Norton, 1967.

Wolberg, Lewis R. (ed.) "Experimental Group: Can They Enhance Adaptation?" Psychiatric Annals, 2:3, March 1972.

8

Family Therapy

Usually, a family is a small group of people tied together by a legal arrangement, sex and/or love, heredity, common goals and/or customs and/or beliefs, for the purposes of self-protection in a hostile world, begetting and raising children, transmitting the subgroup culture, and companionship. Sometimes very few of these elements are present and yet the concept of "family" remains. For our purposes, we will consider any group of people a family who consider themselves to be.

Families differ greatly from one another in the manner in which they are organized, in how effective they are in achieving their purposes, in how flexible they are and how capable of change and in how healthy and prosperous they are. Families differ in their governing principles and may be categorized by the type of rule or who rules as: (1) autocratic, (2) democratic, (3) despotic, (4) patriarchal, or (5) matriarchal. Families differ in their relationships with other families and individuals and range from broadly cosmopolitan to narrowly parochial.

An operating, established family functions like a single organism with various parts, and is often related to and spoken of as being a unit—as being an extended person. "The Smiths are liars. I'd never trust them." "Aren't the Joneses lovely people?" "The Kellys are really quick. You can't pull anything over on them."

THE "DIFFERENT" FAMILY MEMBERS

When one member of a genetically based family differs from the group it does not go unnoticed. "I don't care what they say, Harry just doesn't act like a Robinson. He doesn't even look like one." Or, "I hate to say it, but the kid looks more like Joe than he does like his father."

So, both outside of and within the family, certain expectations develop regarding appearance, behavior, intelligence, deportment, talent, even strength and energy level. Simultaneously pressure develops, again both outside and inside the family, to make all members conform to predictable "family patterns."

Now, since genetics and growth and development are so very complicated and therefore unpredictable in people, it happens quite often that families produce children who are or who become very different from their relatives. Take just one factor, for example, energy level. A quiet, peaceloving, amiable, low-energy family has a hyperkinetic, high-energy youngster who is into everything, asking questions, constantly active. The family is "going out of their minds" with this kid. They love him, even admire his quickness, but it exhausts them "just watching him." Depending on the total family makeup, this "deviant" child (really quite normal) will have various pressures brought to bear by family and friends to conform to the normal energy level of his parents. His response to these pressures will cause other reactions to take place, and in the worst possible situation, the child will become mentally ill or the family will break up, one parent "siding" with the child, the other not.

Let us take another example. A very bright successful couple have a child of just average intelligence. They sensibly decide to give the child every advantage and opportunity to develop to his fullest but agree not to push him to college or to insist that he follow either of their careers. They are disappointed to be sure, but they love their child and vow that they will in no way let him feel inferior because he happens not to be brilliant. So far so good. When this first child is five they have their second baby. The difference in the children is startling. Child number two is far brighter, far more alert and active, holds his head up, crawls, follows objects and does everything much earlier than their first child. There is no question about it; the second child is much more like the parents than the first, and they like the second child much more. Unless the parents are very careful, as well as very imaginative and resourceful, they could easily have problems with both children.

These two examples illustrate how very serious problems can develop in normal families when a child is given them who is somehow "different." The parents in these examples are not mentally ill nor are they heartless monsters. They both face a very difficult, though not uncommon, problem.

Also remember that these examples are very much oversimplified. It hardly ever happens in real life that problems occur in isolation like this. Usually there are several problems going on at the same time in various stages of being solved or of not being solved, such as financial difficulties, troubles with relatives or neighbors, job hassles, illness, sexual or personality conflicts between husband and wife. It is in the midst of all of these that the "different" child appears as in the examples above. Still we have oversimplified. What we have postulated so far is: (1) a "normal" (ordinary) family with (2) ordinary problems into which is born (3) a "different" child. But let us stop at this level of complexity for a moment. This child can have a "problem with adjustment," as they say in schools, and the guidance counselor can call the parents in to explain to them that their child has a problem.

Of course the child has a problem, but perhaps he wouldn't have in a different family. His difficulties developed at home, in his own family, and as long as he is living there, there is going to be *no way* he can learn to adjust to the family unless they learn to adjust to him at the same time. If the child were taken into individual psychotherapy (look back over the two examples) how would you treat him? Would you tell the child in the first example that he should understand that his parents are slower than he is, and he must adjust to this? How does he adjust? By slowing down? By trying to become something other than he is? How about the first born in example number two? Would you tell him that his parents like his younger brother better because he is brighter and more like them? Or would you lie and say the parents liked both children equally? How would you tell your patient he is really an OK person?

As you can see, treating one member of a family group for problems which have arisen out of the group and its feelings and reactions is quite impossible unless that one member has already separated from or intends to separate from the family group. When the member presenting problems is still living with the family, then the family must be treated together in that modification of group therapy that we call *family therapy.*

We have said that our examples remain oversimplified. This is because we have drawn a picture of ordinary parents with ordinary problems. Parents like this are usually willing to acknowledge their role in the child's maladjustment and welcome help in figuring things out as a family unit.

What if one parent is psychotic or alcoholic, or both? What if the mother has multiple sclerosis? What if there is no father in the home at all, and the mother is prostituting to make money to supplement her welfare check because she is addicted to heroin and the kids are actually starving?

This degree of complexity is also seen at a mental health center. In this very last example, although there is a family in trouble, family therapy would hardly be considered. Most likely in this case an attempt would be made to get the mother into the day hospital and place the children in foster home care until the mother could provide a reasonable home for them.

Judgment must be used as to when family therapy is a feasible modality and when it is out of the question.

DEVELOPMENT OF FAMILY THERAPY THEORY

Families are composed of individual members who together form a small group. When individuals develop neurotic symptoms in reaction to unconscious conflict then psychoanalysis, or a modification of it, may be the treatment of choice.

Psychoanalysis is neither quick nor inexpensive as a therapeutic tool. It focuses on the individual, and is not particularly concerned with the patient's family, friends, job, social milieu, ethnic group, etc., except in regard to the patient's feelings about them, and *his* manner of dealing with them. Psychoanalysis focuses on intrapsychic functioning exclusively, and therefore uses a single patient concept. When the family or social group of the individual is disorganized and chaotic, and he reacts by developing neurotic symptoms because he is unable to leave or change his situation it does not seem valid to continue to focus treatment on the intrapsychic process while excluding the external pressures causing the symptoms. The beginning nurse in a community mental health center setting, will hear terms like *psychoanalytically-oriented therapy* and *insight-oriented therapy*, or *intensive one-to-one therapy*, or any variety of terms (see Chapter 1) meant to indicate the individual therapist's modified version of the psychoanalytic technique. This happens, we suppose, because it is difficult to give up old labels. Also, it is reassuring to some therapists to get into heady discussions with their peers about their use of and familiarity with Freudian technique. The fact is that almost no psychotherapist ignores the patient's family situation or social group as genuine sources of pathogenic influence on the individual. In community psychiatric practice it is always considered and frequently dealt with directly.

Family therapy, in retrospect, was a predictable evolution of psychotherapeutic concepts. As a therapy system it represented processive as well as progressive change. At first, only mothers of mentally ill children were considered important, and they were studied. The psychiatrist treated the child, the social worker counselled the mother (on cue from the doctor), the psychologist tested both and the nurse kept her eye on everyone. If the child was diagnosed schizophrenic, then the mother was labeled schizophrenogenic. (Translated, that means the mother is considered the major cause of her child's illness.) Studies described her as insecure, domineering, aggressive, controlling, manipulative and rejecting. Characteristically it was discovered that the relationship between mother and child was intense, and the mother was frequently overprotective in a smothering way. Theorists began to refer to this special type of abnormal mother-child relationship as symbiotic. In its psychiatric sense symbiosis represents the inability of two individuals, such as a mother and child, to separate and to function independently of each other. This mutual dependence does not foster individuation, and effectively curtails emotional growth. It is a pathogenic tie between mother and child.

Later studies examined the father's role in the development of the mother-child relationship. The father was often found to abdicate his parental role, deferring to his wife's judgment and wishes. Such fathers were seen to be ineffective, passive and inadequate. In a sense the child was surrendered to the mother to raise as she saw fit. The pathogenic nature of this position then contributed to the child's blocked development and symptom formation. Today we know that the father's role in the development of the child's personality is vital. Once the baby is born the active presence and participation of the father is necessary if there is to be a true family structure. "The father's involvement determines whether at birth the infant is delivered to a group or merely shifts from biologic to biophysic unity with the mother. Similarly, the father's participation determines the degree of the mother's isolation . . . There must be two parents to provide a stable base and a meaningful group."[1]

It is now accepted theory that all family members exert influences on each other to conform to the collective standards or norms, even if those norms are deviant. Healthy families are flexible and tolerant, encouraging and facilitating individual growth. In contrast, sick families are rigid, fortress-like groups. There is excessive use of censure and reward systems to keep members in line.

Disregard for or breaking of established (but not always defined) family rules brings punishment—banishment or scapegoating. For the "bad" member, being sent away or banished can be preferable to remaining and being the family scapegoat.

Whether the family is healthy or sick, or, as is most often the case, somewhere in between, there is a homeostatic principle on which it operates. Everything is changing, all the time. Life would become impossible unless the biologic process had ways of coping with the fluidity and constancy of change. Plant, animal and human life all have physiologic homeostatic systems which maintain and regulate and monitor reaction to change. When the environment changes radically, and the regulatory systems are overwhelmed, serious danger, even death, can occur. In order to maintain function, and to diminish the danger and discomfort of environmental change, human beings develop compensating systems to maintain homeostasis. If the family encounters or perceives attack it will respond in a way designed to maintain its homeostasis, thereby preserving its function, good or bad. Another principle of family homeostasis is that change in one member effects changes in other family members. Ackerman states that "The matrix of human relationships, whether healthy or sick, is the family; for this reason, the family is the natural point for intervention when the homeodynamic principle breaks down."[2]

In community mental health practice the nurse will frequently encounter family groups in which the ability to cope with the changing, frequently hostile environment is not successful. The family's homeostatic mechanism is either faulty or overwhelmed. This is particularly true with families of adolescent drug users. Also, when families are missing one parent, they become more vulnerable, as the one parent attempts to cope with both parental roles. Add poverty to any of these situations and everything is more difficult. In the case of Mrs. L. (see p. 177) there was essentially healthy family interaction with much support for the mother, but the social pressures faced by the family badly taxed the basic family homeostasis. Mrs. L's depression over her inability to make needed changes in her living situation would surely have effected changes in the behavior of her children if some resolution of her problem had not been possible. In the M case, (see p. 122) the family is sick, and Barry's symptoms clearly cause changes in other family members.

The M family is given as an example because it so graphically demonstrates family pathology and its development over three generations. Also, the family demonstrates the "core concept of family psychotherapy . . . that the mental illness of a member is a symptom or aspect of a greater interlocking family pathology, and . . . the oustanding contribution . . . of family psychotherapy studies has been the elaboration of shared unconscious pathology in families."[3]

To summarize, the basic theoretical concepts of family therapy are:

1. Rejection of the single patient concept.
2. Recognition of the identified patient as symptomatic of family psychopathology.
3. Acknowledgment of the cause and effect relationship between social environment and pressures, and family dynamics.
4. Scapegoating technique, used to keep family members in line, to punish errant members (but usually focused on one member at a time), is a characteristic of pathogenic families.
5. Pathologic double bind—the damned if you do, damned if you don't situation. Particularly disruptive to children and adolescents. Causes feelings of rage, frustration, anxiety, fear and helplessness, and promotes feelings of insecurity.
6. Symbiotic tie refers to a pathogenic relationship between the mother and child. Ego development and individuation of the child is suppressed, while strong identification and dependence on mother is encouraged. (Substitute *smothering* for mothering.)
7. Schizophrenogenic describes the aggressive, domineering, overprotective, "insecure" and rejecting parent. It can describe the mother, the father, or the family collectively. Meant to indicate the pathologic interaction which is both cause and effect in seriously disturbed families.
8. Principle of family homeostasis specifies that both sick and healthy families try to preserve their family system and function. It also specifies that changes occurring in one member will produce change in another. (e.g., in typical family therapy intervention with a psychotic family, it is very common to observe the identified patient's improvement result in decompensation of a "well" family member.
9. Paradoxical communication, typical of pathologic family interaction, involves incongruent but consistent contradic-

tion, qualification, or denial of previously made statements and actions. It results in distrust, confusion, and ultimately meaningless communication, or no communication at all. It can be verbal or nonverbal. (In politics it is described as a *credibility gap.* The public is told "the truth," only to learn later that "truth" was lie. The lie is rationalized to look similar to the original truth. Repetition of this process is confusing, makes the public uneasy, distrustful, suspicious and angry. "Nobody believes politicians anyway, that's just political garbage.")

TECHNIQUE OF FAMILY THERAPY

As previously indicated, the first contact the community mental health nurse may have with a disturbed family may be with the "identified patient." This is so because entire families rarely come for treatment, although mothers and fathers will often decide to seek therapeutic assistance if they have a marital problem. If the couple has children, then the possibility of family therapy should be considered and discussed. Many people reject the idea as unfamiliar, and more frequently as unnecessary. "Our children are fine, the only problems are between us." This may be correct, but the chances that it is are slim. The nurse who suspects, by reason of her assessment of a destructive relationship between the parents, that the children may need an opportunity to get unsqueezed from the family's neurotic or psychotic vise, should indicate her feelings to the parents. She can say with candor, "Well, you say there are no problems between you and your children, but my experience makes me doubt that." If the family system is troubled but not closed and impregnable (as some are), then there is a good chance the family will agree to at least an evaluation interview.

The number of children in the family and their age will affect the decision to include them, and whether to use a co-therapist. If there are toddlers, they may be a distraction during an interview and are likely not to get too much out of therapy. However, if there are several children and they are in pubescence or adolescence they will probably have strong feelings about coming in for treatment. Some will approach it as a challenge ("they won't get me to say anything"), some as an opportunity to let their parents know what they are feeling (and in the process find out things they did not realize about their parents), while others may flatly refuse therapy, as in the M family used as a case example in this chapter. If there are less than three children the therapist may feel comfortable alone, but we recommend a co-therapist in any situation where one or more of the following exist:

1. Two or more children.
2. Inexperience of the therapist.

3. If the sexual distribution of the family is disproportionate (e.g., three daughters, an aggressive mother and a passive father, might be more successfully treated with a male co-therapist).

4. If the family is acutely disturbed, the chaos and disorganization in such situations is incredibly taxing and distracting, even to an experienced therapist. The co-therapist can help share the load, help keep order, and share observations.

In selecting a co-therapist, it is a good idea to know the individual with whom you will be working. It would certainly be undesirable to have disagreements (verbal or nonverbal) about some basic things like sex, social values, etc., likely to be touched on in these family therapy sessions. You should be comfortable with the co-therapist and like the person. It's OK to disagree, an occasional disagreement in front of a family where this is denied or "not allowed" can be a therapy stratagem. It is necessary to find out first what the areas of disagreement are and to make some decisions with your partner about how to handle them in therapy sessions.

In gaining an understanding of the family system two things are necessary: a thorough history concentrating on families of origin and each member's feelings about his "first family," and careful observation of the family patterns of interaction.

It is important to note the communication patterns: who talks to whom, and how? In a family system there may be many dyadic and triadic relationships. Some members are left out. All these things will be quickly apparent to the skilled therapist, but can be learned by the novice. It can be helpful to have the family tape-record their therapy session after you have indentified patterns of paradoxical communication, or other confusing interaction that you want the family to pick up. The tape recorder can be a valuable didactic tool to both the family and the therapist. The family can learn that patterns exist which it has denied; the therapist can check out her impressions and observations, and validate them with a peer or consultant. Most families who make the commitment to come for therapy are anxious to find out what's going on and will readily agree to the use of the tape recorder. However, that does *not* mean the families are agreeing to *change*.

It is an excellent idea to establish some *guidelines* with families. *The authors have found the following useful:*

1. Therapy contract. This should include who attends family sessions, where they will occur (at the community mental health center or in the family home), the fee, the duration of therapy sessions and the length of therapy. We suggest a one to one and one-half hour session once a week for a fixed number of sessions (e.g., 20 or 25 weeks). The temporal limitations should reflect the therapist's estimate of the time needed to achieve whatever goals have been identified.

2. Encourage family members to participate in identifying goals, and remind them that nothing can *make* them change, and your job is *not* to try. The effort must be theirs. Their desire to change will be the motivating force, but will only be facilitated by their ability and determination to do so. You are their expert guide. Therapy really is work, and wishing doesn't make things happen. When this is explained, just as in individual or group therapy, some family member is sure to speak for the family (the family "spokesman") and say something like, "Well then, why the hell should we bother coming here?" The expectation and treasured fantasy is that the therapist will cure, that "The therapist will make things change." There is the hope of magical transformation; the therapist is really a magician! This must be acknowledged by the therapist, and even if it is never voiced openly, be assured it is there. It should be introduced by the therapist if she feels it is lurking in the background. Deal with it directly: "I have the feeling you all expect *me* to make things get right in this family." Pause, someone may respond. If not, continue: "Am I correct? It sure feels to me like that's what everyone is waiting for." There is always some response to this, and if the therapist is lucky and intervenes at the right moment, something unique and significant for the family members and the therapist happens.

3. Ground rules about the content of the sessions: The focus is on the family as a whole entity needing help, not the identified patient. The therapist must clearly state at the beginning that there can be no scapegoating or punishment of the member who takes the risk of telling-it-like-it-really-is, or at least how he thinks it is. There are *family myths*, and they are not to be protected. One goal of therapy is to clarify and discard them. (In the case study of the M family, one myth that Barry challenged was that there were no problems in the family except himself.) Stating that there must be no punishments or prohibitions against revealing family myths does not necessarily prevent that from happening, but it can double bind (in this case the therapeutic double bind) the family members who agree to the rule in the name of getting on with therapy. They may later turn around and try to impose sanctions against the "informer."

4. The family therapist becomes part of the family system. She reaches out and touches, literally and figuratively. By use of self in empathetic response to the family's concerns and struggles she can and should share her own emotions openly and honestly. The therapist sets a model for the family, demonstrating that openness, directness and honest statement of feelings is OK and not dangerous. If, as often happens, the mother or father reveals something about his or her childhood that was painful, and there is no immediate response nor support from the other members, the therapist should feel perfectly free to say how she was affected by the revelation. "That must have been a terrible experience for you, I know it would have been for me. Perhaps that explains why you have been unhappy." The therapist may find other

members reacting with more open support or anger, depending on the situation. The therapist is not a magician, but with her skillful and honest use of self she is a teacher.

5. Allow for some unpredictables. During the course of treatment the family therapist will find it necessary to be a parent figure, a Guru, an advocate, an adversary, an interpreter, an innovator, a provocateur and a conductor. Guidelines are useful only if they enable the nurse to help the family uncover and strip away its crippling pretenses and poses while learning how to reintegrate what it has learned if it decides to move in that direction. The nurse practitioner will find, alone or as a co-therapist, that some families decide not to change, and that is their option.

Some families, or individual members, experience great anxiety and are very threatened as they feel themselves losing control when maladaptive behavior is jettisoned. The nurse should recognize the tension and heightened sense of danger the family feels, and acknowledge it: "I think it is very difficult to give up old ways of doing things. Even if they don't work, they are familiar. It always seems risky to me; even when I feel I want to change, it can scare the hell out of me until I get my bearings." If that is true, and is stated candidly, it can be reassuring. However, the therapist must not be intimidated by this increased anxiety. She cannot be an open, honest, cool and reassuring model while trying to handle her own uncertainty and fear. Just as in work with drug addicts (see Chapter 11, "Drug Addiction and Alcoholism") it is necessary to be very certain of your own feelings (in this case about *your* family) before trying to help others.

SUMMARY:

There are many modifications of therapeutic intervention with disturbed families. It is a new modality, really only accepted in the last decade or so as a valid therapeutic approach. This chapter is meant as an overview, presenting the basic theoretical concepts of family therapy. It is not meant to provide the student with a rundown on in-vogue innovations. Because we could not state it more succinctly, but agree with its content, we quote Framo on the training, learning, and qualities of a therapist.[4]

"Much of what transpires between patients and therapists is expressed by tone, gestures, expression, sensory impressions, feelings, and a host of other almost incommunicable states. Only a small part of therapeutic commerce takes place via words. Therapy supervisors have long known that a wide discrepancy frequently exists between what a therapist says he does and what he actually does do. For example, one therapist may believe he is dealing with very deep material, but its impact on the patient may be quite shallow; another

therapist may believe he is only doing supportive psychotherapy by dealing exclusively with reality problems, yet discover to his astonishment that the patient has become thoroughly involved. A further argument against defining techniques is that all therapists vary widely in personality, style,
amount of activity, quality of focusing, goals, etc., even
within the same psychotherapeutic school. Moreover, no
amount of reading on technique will make an effective psychotherapist. It has long been known, but rarely stated, that
meaningful psychotherapy demands from the therapist the
necessary personality equipment (admittedly difficult to
specify) capable of development under . . . supervision. This
supervision in order to be effective, should take place in a free
'therapeutic' atmosphere which permits exploration of the
feelings of the student."

CASE STUDY—THE M FAMILY

The following case study was selected because it demonstrates all of
the major theoretical concepts of family therapy.

In the case to be discussed the nuclear family consists of a
father, mother, and two sons, aged 17 and 14. The identified
patient was the 17-year-old son, Barry. The family became
known to the community mental health center when Barry
was admitted for evaluation. The admitting information, sup-
plied by the parents, indicated bizarre, erratic and obsessive-
compulsive behavior in the home—primarily focused in the
bathroom where Barry would spend hours (eight or more) at
a time. The history indicated an acute onset of symptoms.
However, after discussion with the family and the patient, it
was easily possible to see that symptoms of acute disturbance
had been present for the past five years. When Barry was 12, a
contact was made with the family service sponsored by the
M's church because of his "uncontrolled temper tantrums."
As a result of this contact a complete psychiatric evaluation
was performed and it was decided that the possibility of
childhood schizophrenia was present. The psychologist, however, on the basis of psychological testing, ruled out schizophrenia "at this time," but indicated a severe adjustment reaction of childhood with a predisposition to schizoid characteristics "unless the parents can be helped to accept this child
as different from others."

(Both evaluations, although in disagreement on specific
diagnosis, agreed that there were patterns of disturbance within the family and that any help to the child would necessarily
include helping the parents. There was accentuated inability

to separate from his mother (symbiosis) and inability to derive any satisfaction in a relationship with his father who admittedly disapproved of, neglected and physically mistreated Barry. Significantly, the father was "completely satisfied" with his younger son—and indicated a preference and "strong feeling" for this son to the exclusion of Barry.)

The interim years had been difficult and barely tolerable according to the parents. Barry was seen in therapy for a brief time with the Family Service psychologist following his contact with them. At that time Barry displayed some insight into his problem, but because he was faced with rejection both within and without his home, from his father as well as his peers, he could only explain that he was "desperately unhappy" and attributed his tantrums to the real situation in which he lived. Because the necessary psychiatric help was denied him and because, as predicted, the abuse continued, Barry had gradually deteriorated emotionally until an acute exacerbation with psychotic reaction was manifested, precipitating his first psychiatric admission.

Discussion of Family Background and Dynamics:

The family appeared to be of lower-middle to middle income. They were a first generation family; both paternal and maternal grandparents were born abroad. High school education was the maximum level attained, although the father had some technical training which enabled him to operate his own T.V. repair business. The parents explained that they had waited three years after their marriage to have Barry, and that his birth was "planned." The father explained that the birth of a son was an occasion of great pride and joy, an opportunity for the son to achieve prominence and thus vicariously satisfy his parents—particularly his father's unsatisfied needs for accomplishment. The mother was an only child whose mother (widowed) lived in an adjoining house with an interconnecting passageway (suggesting a symbiotic tie between the mother and grandmother).

Mrs. M was in her late thirties, verbal, aggressive and critical. She was anxious and concerned about her son but wanted "the doctors to do something." She manifested only superficial insight and was resentful and frequently unaccepting of any suggestion of her role in her son's illness. She made such statements as: "Ask anyone, ask my neighbors. They'll tell you better parents never existed." "Even Barry says he doesn't know what caused his sickness but he knows it's not us." "Well, tell us what we are doing wrong, and we'll correct it!" "Look at Jim (younger son). There's nothing wrong with him. Now I ask you, would a mother or father treat one good and one bad? No!"

The father was slightly older, of medium build, masculine in appearance, and quite tense. He presented an air of resignation and hopelessness about Barry. ("Well, what can be done now?") He also expressed his feelings of hostility, rejection and guilt towards his oldest son. He seemed less defensive than his wife, and during the course of the interview was interrupted and excoriated by her. He seemed willing to take some of the blame but he saw his wife and her mother as also guilty. He was more direct in his comments about Barry and tended to use denial less. A sample of his comments was revealing: "God, that kid (Barry) can make me so mad! Sometimes I just have to leave the house or I'm afraid I'll kill him." "Barry's trouble is that he feels inferior. Jim excels in everything, Barry is the complete opposite." "I never had any time to spend with him (Barry) for the first three years; after that it was too late. I've wanted to be a pal to him—take him to a ball game or something like that but he's not interested in sports like Jim and me. I don't know what went wrong—I guess I let him down."

Jim, the 14-year-old brother, was an attractive, pleasant, articulate youngster who seemed to have genuine regard and feelings for his brother, but who had become impatient with the "tricks Barry pulls and gets away with." He was ambivalent about Barry. He admitted that he liked Barry but was embarrassed by Barry's behavior and aspirations which he considered unsatisfactory. Jim had some obvious difficulties himself; he was moderately obese and it appeared that his weight problem was recent. In family discussion the interaction between Jim and his father was stronger and more supportive than the interaction between Jim and his mother. Thus Jim would comment on his father's self-criticism of his role in Barry's illness, "Gee Dad, it isn't all your fault. Barry does egg you on—I think he really asks for it." He explained his analysis of Barry's problems and his reaction to Barry: "The trouble with Barry is he doesn't have any friends. He never got along good with the other guys—and he was left out of everything. He isn't interested in sports like my friends and my Dad and me. A guy needs friends. Myself—I have lots of friends, I get along good with the other kids. Everyone makes fun of Barry—and that really bugs me, but Barry really invites it. (How?) Well—he wears his pants too high up on his waist and it makes him walk funny, y'know—not like a guy should walk. And then he wears his sports shirts with the top button buttoned! None of the other guys wear them like that. Now his other problem is that he isn't going to college. He's getting older now (17) and he's going to find out that he made a mistake, and then he'll really be mad at himself."

"I get mad at him—he, oh, I don't know! (Embarrasses you?) Yeah—he embarrasses me! Not much, but I guess I'd like to be able to look up to him and the truth is I can't. It makes me mad at him. Another thing he does too—the way he acts towards my Dad—he shouldn't treat Dad so mean—he curses at him and stuff like that." Jim's comments regarding his mother were less tolerant: "Gee Mom, you let Barry get away with murder!"

The interactions of this family suggest a cleavage: father and son against mother and son. Family interaction is disturbed, and this disturbance is sustaining and nurturing to Barry's identified illness, as well as to the pathologic process this family uses to relate to each other. In addition to the two symbiotic patterns already identified there is a probable other, between mother and grandmother. This relationship is perceived by the husband as a threat: "Barry's always been babied by my wife and her mother—*they* made a sissy out of him!" "My wife and her mother are very close—maybe they are too close."

The existence of these coalitions is significant, and within the disturbed family process necessary. They are symbiotic systems and although in conflict with each other they function because of each other.*

The parents were married 21 years ago. The father had returned from the service and struggled during the first few years of the marriage with the multi-adjustments to marriage, civilian life, technical studies and the oppressiveness of a too close relationship between his wife and her mother. After three years of marriage a carefully planned pregnancy occurred and the hoped-for son, Barry, was born. The father stated with feeling, "My God, a son, I remember how proud I was." The mother recalled: "After such a wait it was good. I was sort of lonely. Barry was good company, and you know my husband was never home." Barry's arrival filled many needs for his parents—*and* his grandparents who lived next door.

---

*Symbiotic involvements in the family are more complex than ordinarily considered: they always involve a third party who is essential for the maintenance of the system . . . emphasis has shifted from the concept of the pathogenic parent to the pathogenic family relationship, usually encompassing . . . the nuclear family group . . . Among the possible causes of schizophrenia is . . . a disturbed marital relationship in the parents . . . and grandparents of the patient. This . . . can be viewed . . . in the pathologic mother-child symbiosis (which) has some of its origin in a prior series of unsatisfactory marital relationships: that of the mother to her husband and that of the mother's mother to her husband. This three-generation concept seems an important contribution arising from the study of family pathology."[5]

The father remembered that his wife and mother-in-law "babied him, they kept him in a crib too long, never let him do anything." The mother resented these criticisms and rationalized that because she was an only child her son meant a great deal to her parents. Also, she recalled that her father paid attention to Barry—which her husband never did.

During the first three years Barry was the only recipient of much maternal attention. His father was not present or significant to him at this time. The role model which Barry needed in order to develop a concept of his own masculine identity was absent. In his fourth year Barry suffered three traumas, two overt and one covert. Within one month his mother gave birth to a new brother, his grandfather died, and his father reacted in a warm, receptive and loving way to the new baby while ignoring Barry. Barry, by his father's admission, was neglected by him in favor of Jim. The father recalled that he "sensed something different" about Barry. He found Barry was not "all boy," not the son he had hoped for. He felt also that Barry "*belonged* to his mother and grandmother." The father's joy at having a second son is equatable with having a second chance. He was determined to win the affection of the newest son. In essence he shifted his regard and aspirations for Barry to Jim. The mother settled for this arrangement. She recalled that she was glad that her husband paid so much attention to Jim; Barry could remain "her baby." (Significantly, Barry today addresses his parents as Mommy and Daddy, while his younger brother calls them Mom and Dad.) The nonverbal pact reached was that the mother could continue to develop her symbiotic tie with Barry and the father was free to develop a similar relationship with Jim.

Although the mother stated her marriage has never been bothered with any "real problems—except Barry" evidence seemed to contradict her. It is probable that the marital relationship had not been satisfying to the parents.

During the second family session when the subject of the M's "perfect except for Barry" marriage came up, Barry alone protested by screaming out loud, "That's a lie." Mrs. M, Mr. M and Jim shook their heads negatively in response to Barry's outburst. Barry immediately gave ground. The development of the symbiotic pattern between the mother and Barry can be seen as directly related to the father's reaction to it. If he chose he could have penetrated it, but by rejection, indifference and isolation it was intensified and supported. Instead, he attempted to build a similar, although less intense and less dangerous, relationship with his youngest son.

As Barry developed it became apparent that he was "different." He manifested problems of obesity and dysplastic body habitus with an unusual shape to his head at the temporal mandibular area bilaterally, and increased angulation of the hip joint which caused him to walk in a peculiar feminine fashion. Because of these physical characteristics, which he could neither help nor change, he became the victim of unending taunts and jokes. He was beaten by his peers as well as his father, and his sense of rejection and worthlessness was acute. He was called "queer" and "faggot," and his masculinity was questioned constantly by his father who told Barry that the beatings he administered were because the child was a "coward" and a "sissy." His mother recalled "when his father beat him I feared for his life, that's how bad it was —and still is!"

Speculation about the father's abuse of his son involved the use of two mechanisms: 1) guilt: This feeling grew within him because of the early neglect and rejection of the boy which he expiated in a complex, pathologic manner by first projecting it onto the child; 2) identification: The father saw Barry as effeminate, passive, and putty in his mother's hands in much the same way as he felt, so that by punishing Barry's submissiveness and weakness he was also punishing his own passivity—the son being an extension of the father.

As a result of abuse from his father and peers Barry regressed to a less threatening level of emotional development, and increased the symbiotic bond with his mother in which he sought refuge. The father was then able to justify his close relationship with Jim as a compensation for his dissatisfaction and failure with Barry. Jim responded to this demand, probably because he sensed too great a danger in a close relationship with his mother.

The interaction described had never been healthy, always pathologic. The help that Barry should have received during past years was not provided and Barry had decompensated during the interim.

Predictably, the mother and Barry were the most resistant to therapy. The mother stated, "Barry is the one who is sick, not us." Barry attributed his "problems" to an "upset stomach" and asked "Do I look crazy?" The methodology and philosophy of family therapy were explained and questions were provoked so that a more receptive attitude to the intervention could be encouraged. However, despite these precautions and the family's acute need, therapy was discontinued after two sessions when Mrs. M called to inform the therapist that she had placed Barry in a private mental hospital.

The therapist working with the M family was experienced in family therapy theory and had much clinical experience. But the family's pathology was so rigidly defended by the members that there was no breaking into their system. Maintaining their sick homeostasis required Barry's continued identification as the patient, and Barry was a willing, cooperative participant.

REFERENCES

1. Forrest, T. "The Paternal Roots of Male Character Development." Psychoanalytic Rev., 55 (2):83, 1967.
2. Ackerman, N. W. "Family Therapy." *In* S. Arieti (ed.), The American Handbook of Psychiatry, Vol. III, New York: Basic Books, 1966. p. 203.
3. Borzormenyi-Nagy, I., Framo, J.L. et al. Intensive Family Therapy. New York: Harper and Row, 1965. p. 23.
4. *Ibid.*, p. 144.
5. *Ibid.*, pp. 19-23.

FURTHER READING

Minuchin, S., Montalvo, B., Guerney, B., Rosman, B. and Schumer, F. Families of the Slums. New York: Basic Books, 1967.
Satir, V. Conjoint Family Therapy. Palo Alto, California: Science and Behavior Books, 1967.
Watzlawick, P., Beavin, J. and Jackson, D. Pragmatics of Human Communication. New York: W. W. Norton, 1967.

9

Partial Hospitalization— The Day Hospital

CASE I

Margaret McS had spent 20 of her 45 years in institutions, first being hospitalized at the age of 15. Her pattern after release from the state hospital was to return for medication followup for three or four months, then stop her drugs, gradually become psychotic again and be returned to the hospital about one year after her release.

This time, the center's emergency service responded to a call from Mrs. McS's landlady, and on a home visit found Mrs. McS sitting on the floor of her tiny room, humming and singing to herself, rocking back and forth, her hair and the entire room caked with feces mixed with food. The home visit team brought her directly to the day hospital where she was showered and put in clean clothes. She was medicated and she attended group therapy. By day's end it was felt that she could best be handled in the inpatient unit for several days, because she was still too confused to travel alone and her landlady refused to have her back. However, all of the beds were filled. There were no other hospitals available because she was not technically an emergency (overtly dangerous to herself or others). With the assistance of another patient, temporary living arrangements were made and within three weeks Mrs. McS had her own place again in another rooming house. Special care was taken in planning the followup so that Mrs. McS would not slip again into her usual pattern. It has now been three years since this episode, the longest period she has had outside of the hospital since she was 15. Once each month she returns to the day hospital for two days whether she needs it or not. If she does not come in on her own a home visit is made at once.

CASE II

On July 15th, John B was arrested at 2:00 a.m. on a complaint by neighbors that he was prowling down the back alley stark naked with a pillowcase over his shoulder and a flashlight. The police found a dead cat in the pillowcase. He was booked for public indecency and suspicious behavior and jailed until morning. At 9:00 a.m. the police brought him to the emergency service of the center and by 10:30 a.m. he was attending group therapy in the day hospital. Charges were dropped by the police in August. On September 1st he returned to work driving a milk truck and began treatment in the evening hospital two evenings a week. November 5th he was discharged from the program.

CASE III

Tim B was 18 when he finished his first year of college with a 4.0 average and went to California to work for the summer. While there he got deeply involved in mysticism and L.S.D. He withdrew from all social relationships and refused to eat, spending his days and nights walking about dressed only in a long Dashiki reciting poems he had written to no one in particular.

The family Tim was visiting became alarmed and called his father on the East Coast who flew out at once and brough him home. Tim arrived at the center accompanied by hi father, his mother, his older brother, the brother's wife and his uncle Robert B, an attorney in town.

This formidable group descended upon the nurse in the emergency service demanding immediate hospitalization for Tim. After a short time, with everyone in the room talking at once, the nurse asked them all to wait outside while she interviewed Tim alone. Tim began by saying, "They're right. I'm going crazy. If I'm not locked up I'll kill somebody." Then he wept. By the end of the interview the nurse concluded that: (1) Tim was indeed psychotic; (2) his high pressure family was exactly what he didn't need at this time; (3) he wasn't in any way dangerous to himself or others; and (4) he needed immediate treatment.

She took Tim directly to the day hospital and explained the situation to the staff, then returned to deal with the rest of the family. When they heard her decision of partial hospitalization they violently opposed it. Tim couldn't live at home because he was crazy and because the neighbors would find out and it would ruin the father's business. If he "ran away to California again" the family would sue the center and the nurse for malpractice. How could a nurse make these decisions anyway? Where was the doctor? Where was the head of the center? Did the nurse know what would happen when Senator P called the Commissioner of Mental Health in the morning? Uncle Robert left to make a telephone call. Mother and father began blaming each other for bringing Tim to a "clinic" instead of a "top drawer" place.

When the nurse felt she had a fairly good picture of the workings of the B family she called the day hospital psychiatrist and asked him to join the meeting. He did. The tone of the conversation immediately became more respectful but still with a distinctly hostile edge. "Doctor, have you seen Tim?" "Yes, I have." "Don't you agree that he is a very sick boy." "I'd call him a young man but I agree he's pretty troubled right now." "Troubled? He's out of his mind. Are you going to put him in the hospital?" "Not right away. Not if we can avoid it. He has already been started on a major tranquilizer and is receiving treatment right now. As soon as we find him a place to stay for the night I think we'll be all set." "A place to stay? Where? What's wrong with a hospital? Why not put him somewhere safe?" "Well, I happen to completely agree with the nurse here. We want to relate to Tim's healthy mature part, not his childish sick part. If we take away his freedom it's like saying 'most of you is a child needing protection and we're going to take over your life.' We want to give him a different message. We are saying to him 'you're really a good guy but you've gotten yourself messed up a bit. You'll be able to make it but you'll need the medicine and we want you to come in here every day for a while until you get things together.' He'll probably do fine." "Probably? You mean you're taking a chance with him out of the hospital?" "Yes."

The next day both the senator and the Commissioner of Mental Health called the doctor. Tim's treatment in the day hospital continued uninterrupted.

Three months later Tim began art school by day and drove a taxi by night. He was happy for the first time in years. He visited his family once for a weekend and returned disorganized and confused. He decided not to visit again.

DISCUSSION

Inpatient Vs. Partial Hospitalization

These three cases are typical of the patients who can be handled by a partial hospitalization service. There are very few persons indeed who cannot be taken directly into a well-functioning day hospital after being seen by the emergency service. A nearby, accessible inpatient unit is necessary as a backup for those who are totally unmanageable in a day setting, but it is needed very seldom. Ten years ago, however, all three of these patients would have certainly been committed to a psychiatric hospital. To commit a person is to remove his freedom, to detach him suddenly from his family and community, to give him a legal record as having had a "psychiatric hospitalization,"* to curtail his sex life, to officially establish (in his mind and others) that he is seriously ill and to invite him to regress and to become dependent on the institution. When the situation is sufficiently dangerous or difficult, hospitalization must absolutely be considered, but the harmful aspects of it must be weighed in the balance against the benefits.

Among the considerations that are *not sufficient reason* to lock a person up are these: (1) bizarre behavior; (2) a suicide attempt; (3) a homicidal threat or behavior; (4) severe degree of depression or psychosis; (5) desire to remove patient from the family; (6) no place to sleep; (7) anxiety of the staff; (8) the psychiatrist wants some rest, or is going away for the weekend; (9) misuse of drugs; and (10) patient's desire to be committed.

Admittedly all of these considerations bring hospitalization to mind. Certainly any of them should be taken seriously. But not at their face value—not without close scrutiny.

Bizarre Behavior

This is always socially determined. What is considered bizarre in one generation or country may not be so considered in another. A patient showing this manifestation is acting against the social norm for *his* time and place. If he is living in a small community he will soon be known as the "town nut." In a large city he will have a lot of company and often go unnoticed. There is generally nothing dangerous about bizarre behavior and it usually clears up rapidly with medication unless it is a very well established chronic symptom. The loss of stature in a community that a person will suffer by being allowed to remain at large must be weighed against the loss of stature resulting from having been in a mental hospital. Also, the possibility of having the patient live away from his own community (but not in a hospital) until his behavior becomes more ordinary must be investigated. An example of bizarre behavior would be the man with the dead cat in the bag or the woman with a postpartum psychosis who carries a doll around with her. The public reaction to this type of behavior is to "lock them up." It is our responsibility as professionals to do the best thing for the patient, all things considered.

---

*Psychiatric hospitalization is, in many states, sufficient ground for removal of a driver's licence or reason to deny a patient certain types of employment. These side effects can have a far more damaging effect on a person's life than the mental illness itself.

Suicide Attempt

Attempted suicide is traditionally considered a reason for inpatient hospitalization. In some patients the "suicide attempt" is not a real danger to their life but serves some other purpose, such as giving leverage for the manipulation of a spouse. This is not to say that such "gestures" are not sometimes accidentally lethal, for they are. The patient coming to the center after such an attempt, however, has usually "made her point," at least for the time being, and it is quite safe to treat her in the day hospital. (Many, in fact, do not even need this intensity of treatment and will do well on a straight outpatient basis.)

On the other hand, inpatient hospitalization is certainly no guarantee against successful suicide. Anyone with a few years experience in psychiatric nursing will recount a case she knew where the patient killed himself while on strict suicide precautions on a locked ward.

Each case of attempted suicide must be assessed individually in terms of the possibility of a recurrence, what the attempt means and what an inpatient setting vs. day hospitalization means to the patient. Some people have such a blatant authority problem that they will redouble their efforts to kill themselves if they are locked up.

Along with the individual case assessment the family, neighbors, friends and other available "community supports" must be taken into consideration. Properly used, these supports can be a powerful deterrent to repetition of a suicide attempt.

Homicidal Threat or Behavior

Most cases of homicide involve someone in the patient's family, as husband killing wife or parent killing child. Most cases of homicide occur in a psychotic or near-psychotic state, aided by alcohol or drugs. In most cases of homicide or attempted homicide, the patient is in no way dangerous immediately after the event, but is subdued, remorseful, guilt-ridden or amnesic about the event. Most cases of this type are jailed with high bail set because they are considered dangerous. From time to time they are released on bail and seek psychiatric evaluation and treatment. There is rarely the need for inpatient hospitalization in this situation. The day hospital is the place of choice. That the other patients will get upset by such a person (a murderer) in their therapy group goes without saying. In our experience however, this has a more devastating effect in a closed setting than in an open one.

Severe Depression or Psychosis

The severity of impairment alone can in no way serve as an indication for one treatment modality or another. A person who is profoundly depressed with severe psychomotor retardation *can* be treated in the day hospital if he can be gotten in on a daily basis, and medication begun at once and monitored continuously. As the depression lightens, the suicidal potential often increases, as the patient then has the energy to do what he had been thinking all along. This is taken into account and the patient is watched carefully both at home and at the center.

Severe psychosis can be treated in the day hospital *unless* the patient is repeatedly combative or assaultive and cannot be contained by medication after a reasonable trial, or his psychosis is such that he is too confused to safely come to the center each day. These exceptions apply to only one or two percent of severely psychotic patients seen on intake.

Removal of Patient From Family

Mental disorder rarely occurs in an isolated individual but rather in a family or social setting where many people contribute to the illness that appears in the patient. When possible, such an interrelated group should be taken into treatment together (see Chapter 8, "Family Therapy."). When this is not possible, the next best thing is often to remove the patient from the pathologic setting. Examples of this are the depressed wife of an alcoholic husband (either may be the patient and profit from being away from the other) and the confused teenager with a domineering, overprotective mother. Before the advent of the community mental health center, such need for separation was usually handled by using an inpatient facility as a temporary retreat. Today, the need for separation of the members in a pathologic grouping is no less than before but is handled by using community resources other than a psychiatric inpatient unit. Hotel rooms, the "Y," boarding and rooming houses are all employed to avoid hospitalization and to accomplish the goal of separation when required.

With a well-functioning partial hospitalization program and a housing coordinator, it is never necessary to consider inpatient hospitalization to "remove a patient from his family."

Homeless Patient

Many patients arrive at the center "without a place to sleep" that night along with whatever other troubles they have. Although this too has been a reason in the past for hospitalization, it is no longer a valid one. Occasionally patients who are attending the day hospital suddenly become homeless, "My husband kicked me out," "My mother said I couldn't stay home any longer." It is not always easy to find satisfactory lodgings for people who are mentally ill on very short notice but it can be done. There is no reason to hospitalize someone because he is homeless.

Staff Anxiety

Staff anxiety in a day hospital, especially in a newly organized one where most of the workers received their training in an inpatient facility, can be a factor weighting decisions in favor of commitment. Experience and programmed staff development will greatly help personnel to deal with their anxiety and to see viable options to hospitalization.

Psychiatrist Not Available

In the past, patients were occasionally placed in mental hospitals "for safety's sake" when their psychiatrist went away on vacation or planned to leave town for a weekend. With the changing delivery system of mental health services, the psychiatrist is no longer central to the treatment of the patient and indeed, less and less central to the mental health team. Many people relate to the patient. Although one person may come to have more importance to a particular patient than the others on the team, there is not that "all-or-none" feeling of one patient and one doctor that is so shattering when it breaks down. Patients are never committed to the hospital when their mental health therapist (of whatever discipline) is not available.

Drug Misuse

Drug misuse is not sufficient reason for mental hospitalization for several reasons. (1) Almost all inpatient settings have illicit drugs available regardless of security precautions that are taken. (2) In the absence of emotional disorder (see Chapter 10, "Medical Problems that Mimic or Complicate Emotional Disorders"), it is inappropriate to treat drug misuse on an inpatient ward. (3) Detoxification should be undertaken on a special unit designed for that purpose with full medical as well as psychiatric coverage. (4) Except for detoxification, the day hospital can provide all of the care of the inpatient unit to the drug misuser.

Drug misuse should, almost without exception, be treated first in the partial hospital where motivation and personality strengths can be evaluated.

Patient Desires Commitment

There are still patients around today who have been trained by the system to expect, even to desire, hospitalization when they begin to feel ill. They need to be retrained to come to the center for help but it is often difficult to get across to them that "20 years ago we told you that the best possible treatment for you was in the state hospital. Now we're telling you that the best possible treatment for you is at home, in your own community."

Small wonder that patients get confused. The fact remains that criteria for hospitalization have changed radically and some people are left with expectations that can no longer be met as they were before.

Of course, a patient's desire for commitment is always heard as possibly containing a warning, a need for control and structure, a fear of imminent personality dissolution. This is an important communication. It is just not by itself sufficient reason for hospitalization.

DAY HOSPITAL MILIEU

What happens in the day hospital? How can so many people be safely handled there who formerly would have needed commitment? Does the staff use some kind of magic that nobody writes about?

The kind of day hospital described in this chapter does use a kind of "magic" that nobody writes about. To really feel it and understand it, it is necessary to work in such a setting. The atmosphere is optimistic and infectious. After the center has been in operation for a period of time a distinctive milieu emerges with certain expectations. It is expected that, once in the day hospital; the patient will get better quickly; he will feel safe and protected there; he will not regress or become more psychotic; appropriate medication will be administered at once and promptly changed when necessary; the capacity for health is within the patient and is about to manifest itself; the staff considers the patient and themselves as important partners in the process of getting better, and that the patient will not be allowed to just walk away from the partnership; hospitalization will be considered only as a last resort because it is far healthier if the patient's strengths can be immediately mobilized to keep him out; and finally, the spouse, children, relatives and neighbors will also be enlisted as partners in the treatment if necessary to keep the patient safely in the community.

Intake procedures, initial interview, financial data and the many necessary written forms are all completed by the emergency service prior to the patient being brought to the day hospital. When the patient arrives with the intake worker, a short verbal report is given to a day hospital staff member in front of the patient.

"Charlie here is kinda messed up, Sue. He took a handful of Elavil last night that he got from his doctor and got pumped out in the accident ward. His wife left him because he was drinking and he hasn't worked for six months. He needs a place to stay tonight and I suspect he's still pretty suicidal. Here are the papers on him. I told him that you people could help him get things together and that he probably wouldn't have to go to the hospital. OK? Charlie, this is Sue Jones. She'll take care of you."

The patient is immediately taken into the program. If it is time for group therapy the patient is started in a group which seems appropriate. The groups are usually heterogeneous and the one with the fewest members will be chosen. Occasionally some groups develop a distinctive characteristic like a "discharge group" or a "young drug takers' group" in which case the choice takes this into consideration.

As soon as there is some time, the practical aspects of the patient's life are quickly explored and handled. If he needs money for a meal or a room it is given or loaned to him. If eligible he is sent or taken to the Department of Public Assistance to apply for welfare. Someone may be assigned to go home with him or to spend the evening with him. A relative or neighbor may be called or asked to come in and take him home if this seems appropriate.

As soon as possible after admission a nurse and psychiatrist take a drug history and prescribe or dispense medication for him for a day or several days.

He is introduced to several patients, some who are well enough to help him and show him around, and some who he may be asked to help.

He is started in the workshop, or placed on the committee to shop for food for tomorrow's lunch, or asked to pitch in and help straighten up a room.

While there are daily staff meetings, the staff concerned about a new patient will have frequent short conversations during his first day to compare their impressions as to whether or not he will "make it." If there is any real worry about this issue they ask for consultation with the director or psychiatrist who will talk with the patient and the staff together and assist with the decision-making process.

Usually, by the end of the first day, the patient has done more things, talked to more people and received more massive support to become healthy than he has in many years. Because the approach is future and health oriented, with the pathology deemphasized, the patient often feels that he didn't get a chance to talk all about his bad experiences and after a few days or weeks discovers that no one will listen anyway. Now, instead, people (staff and patients) continually bombard him with questions about what he is doing and what his plans are, turning his attention to his future and health. As soon as he begins talking about his plans, people begin to ask "When?"

He is taught about his illness from a very particular point of view focusing on his own responsibility. Both depression and psychosis are seen as tending to recur. The treatment is primarily medical (drugs). His responsibility is to recognize the next episode as early as possible and return for treatment at once. He is told that a structured, gratifying, busy life is the best insurance policy against future episodes, and that he has the ability and responsibility to manage this.

PARTIAL HOSPITAL ELEMENTS

Throughout this discussion "day hospital" has been used interchangeably with "partial hospital" for the reason that almost all partial hospitalization programs today still consist only of a day hospital. The next logical element to grow out of the day hospital is the "evening-weekend" hospital. Using the same physical space and facilities as the day program, the evening hospital is ideally suited for patients who have terminated the day program to return to work or school, or for those whose beginning illness has not yet interrupted their usual daytime activities. Two evenings per week is about optimum so that two programs, each with a different focus, can easily take place. For example, a Monday/Wednesday program for chronically ill patients who are suffering an acute exacerbation and need twice-a-week therapy, and a Tuesday/Thursday program for acutely ill patients who are able to continue their usual activity while receiving evening treatment.

By legal definition, one day of partial hospitalization equals six hours of care and one-half day equals three hours. The Department of Public Assistance and offices of mental health generally pay for 120 days (or half days) of partial hospital care. For these reasons, partial hospitals have evolved so that the day hospital often operates from 9:00 a.m. to 3:00 p.m. Monday through Friday, the evening hospital from 6:00 p.m. to 9:00 p.m. Monday through Thursday and the Saturday program from 9:00 a.m. to 3:00 p.m. on Saturday. The times can and do vary from place to place but those given are average. The 120 days (this limit may vary from state to state) can be used up at the rate of five per week, which equals 24 weeks or about a half a year of intensive treatment. This is ample to care for most patients.

FURTHER READING

Glasscote, Raymond M., et al. Partial Hospitalization For the Mentally Ill: A Study of Programs and Problems. Washington, D.C.: The Joint Information Service, 1969, pp. 1-41.

10

Medical Problems That Mimic or Complicate Emotional Disorders

INTRODUCTION

In this chapter we will discuss various physical disorders that present as emotional problems but in which a diagnosable medical illness, measurable by ordinary clinical means, is likely to be missed unless it is considered specifically. *These disorders all cause* **organic** *brain syndrome, or organic brain disease.*

Autopsy studies in state hospitals have revealed an astounding number of cases of organic brain disease that could account for the bizarre behavior of the patient in life, many of which, if diagnosed, could have been treated. Syphilis, "the great pretender," is making a comeback. True to its sobriquet of several generations ago, it can and does mimic every form of emotional illness. Reactions to drugs, notably the hallucinogens and amphetamines, are often indistinguishable from emotional disorders.

The psychiatric nurse should be thoroughly familiar with these conditions and constantly on guard against being lulled into a nonmedical frame of mind by nonnursing colleagues at the mental health center.

On the other hand, the medical-surgical nurse will find her psychiatric experience of great value in the general hospital or clinic where colleagues may be accustomed to disregarding mental symptoms until they become florid and unmanageable.

Any illness that affects a person affects every aspect of that person's functioning. Until recently, most illnesses that presented mentally had almost unmeasurable physical manifestations, and those that presented physically had unmeasurable or unnoticed mental manifestations. This is no longer the situation. Research into biofeedback (alpha wave control) and techniques of meditation, both of which are mental endeavors, has shown conclusively that these have vast and profound measurable physical effects. Similarly, physical endeavors and manifestly physical illnesses have a distinct and measurable mental effect. The nurse is well advised to ask herself with every patient seen, "What are the physical and what are the mental manifestations of this illness?"

As mentioned elsewhere (see p. 86), the treatment of choice in psychosis and depression, the two most common major mental disorders seen, is chemotherapy—medical treatment. Increasing evidence supporting this empiric treatment choice leads us to consider that the predisposition to develop schizophrenia and depression may well be an inherited trait, biochemically measurable.

GENERAL DIAGNOSTIC CONSIDERATIONS

Organic brain syndromes are those conditions in which psychiatric symptomatology is caused by some impairment to the functioning of the brain due to infection, tumor, trauma, toxins or disorders of metabolism or nutrition.

Most of these conditions can be diagnosed by history and physical examination. Some, however, can masquerade as purely functional (mental or psychologic) disorders for a long enough time for the patient to be denied appropriate treatment while the mental health center or other social agencies futilely try all measures available to them to bring about improvement in the condition.

The nurse is not expected to make a detailed differential diagnosis in every case. She should, however, know when to suspect the possibility of an organic brain condition so that referral can be made for the appropriate medical workup. Diseases usually seen in the general hospital rather than in the community mental health center are not discussed in detail here. Examples are postsurgical or posttraumatic psychosis and postencephalitic conditions. When delirium accompanies the prodromal phase of an acute infectious disease, the cause is almost always quite clear when the rest of the symptomatology appears, and would not be subject to misdiagnosis and improper treatment in the community mental health center for very long.

An organic brain syndrome may be acute (short-lived and usually self-terminating—such as drug reactions) or chronic (long-lasting and often causing permanent damage—such as lead poisoning and brain tumor). These are called "acute brain syndrome" and "chronic brain syndrome," respectively.

Any physical symptoms characteristic of neurologic disorders should suggest referral for medical workup, regardless of the nature of the psychiatric complaints. Examples would be headache, convulsions, lapses of consciousness, disorders of gait, vision or speech, weakness, wasting, uncoordination and changes in sensation.

Signs and Symptoms of Organic Brain Syndrome

Mental signs and symptoms that immediately suggest the possibility of an organic brain syndrome, even in the absence of physical symptoms, are the following. They are most important to know.

1. *Any disorder of memory, attention, or orientation.* Both recent memory ("What did you do yesterday?") and remote memory ("Where did you spend your childhood?") should be checked. Inability to pay attention during the interview, forgetting the question, or changing the subject should be noted. Orientation is usually checked in these spheres: *time* ("What is the date today: the month, year, season?"), *place* ("Where are we now? What city and state is this? Where do you live? What is this building?") and *person* ("Who am I? Who is that?").

2. *Emotional liability* (instability). This includes easy crying or laughing throughout the interview or sudden shifts in emotional expression that may or may not be reflective of feelings which are appropriate to what the patient is saying. This symptom is important even when it is reported as a lifelong characteristic.

3. *History or evidence of a sudden change in personality or character.* Examples of this are a normally calm and polite person becoming suddenly rude and irritable, or a law-abiding citizen suddenly beginning to steal and lie, or the sudden appearance of a change in sexual habits.

Coexistence of Organic and Functional Conditions

The possibility of the coexistence of organic and functional conditions must also be considered. A person with depression and anxiety can develop a brain tumor, or the development of an organic brain disease can cause previously hidden psychiatric symptoms to show themselves.

Natural History of the Disease

In addition to the above physical and mental indications of an organic condition, the nurse is aided by a knowledge of the natural history of the ordinary psychiatric disorders, gained by experience. The student will hear and soon begin to make such comments as, "This isn't like an ordinary depression," and "The other schizophrenics I've seen were different from this." When you begin to have these thoughts, allow the possibility of an organic brain syndrome to come to mind.

SPECIFIC CONDITIONS CAUSING ORGANIC BRAIN SYNDROME

Neurosyphilis

Syphilis may be acquired at any age, even from the mother *in utero*. It has been found in proper puritan ladies and clerics of all denominations, as well as in more ordinary citizens. The time lapse between the start of the infection and psychiatric symptoms ranges between three and 40 years. The mental symptoms may appear as a psychoneurosis, a manic-like illness, schizophrenia or depression. Over half, however, show signs of poor judgment, memory defects or euphoria, occasionally with expansive delusions of grandeur. Physical symptoms, when present, include a speech defect with hesitation and slurring (ask the patient to say "Methodist Episcopal"); pupillary changes such as irregularity, inequality or the classic Argyll Robertson pupil which reacts to accommodation but not to light; handwriting disorders with misspelled words, omissions, misplaced or repeated letters and syllables (which the patient does not recognize); changes in the deep tendon reflexes, either increased or diminished; convulsive disorders. Physical stigmata of *congenital* syphilis, when they appear, include Hutchinson's teeth (pegged and/or notched median incisors) and nerve deafness.

The presence of any of these physical signs and symptoms, regardless of the psychiatric symptomatology, should warrant a complete medical workup. The combination of these with judgment or memory defects or expansive thinking ("I own Australia") makes it imperative to rule out syphilis as soon as possible.

Unfortunately, few psychiatric facilities do routine serologies (except on inpatient admission) and only examine the cerebral spinal fluid after a neurologist determines that it should be done. The nurse needs to uncover only one case due to her vigilance to justify her central role on the mental health care team. In crisis intervention and home visiting the nurse may be the "team" all by herself. In neurosyphilis, recovery from all symptoms is often possible with prompt treatment.

Drug and Poison Intoxication

Intoxication is seen fairly frequently by the community nurse. When the causative agent is known there is little immediate diagnostic or treatment problem. A coexistent functional mental illness, if present, will show itself in time. However, when the intoxicating substance is not known (as when the patient will not admit to taking anything because he is suspicious or realistically fears arrest), or when several drugs have been taken at once (which is more and more often the case) a great problem may exist in both diagnosis and treatment. When the symptoms of intoxication are severe and drugs are suspected but not known hospitalization is usually indicated. The patient can then be observed and any untoward effects of treatment measures can be more readily handled.

SEDATIVE INTOXICATION

Intoxication from barbiturates, Doriden, Placidyl, Quaalude and other sedatives resembles simple alcohol intoxication with silly behavior, slurred speech and uncoordinated movements. However, there is no evidence of alcohol on the breath unless the patient has also been drinking. Where these substances have been used chronically, they represent one of the most serious psychiatric/medical emergencies seen today. Abrupt withdrawal can result in convulsions and death.

"Automatic" consumption of sedatives while in a drowsy state may result in accidental overdosage (often mistakenly called a "suicide attempt"). The combination of sedatives and alcohol is frequently lethal.

Sedative usage often coexists with underlying depression or anxiety states and occasionally with schizophrenia.

HALLUCINOGEN INTOXICATION
(Psychotomimetic Intoxication)

L.S.D. (d-lysergic acid diethylamide), D.E.T. (diethyltryptamine), D.M.T. (dimethyltryptamine), D.O.M., or S.T.P. (2, 5-dimethoxy-4-ethyl-amphetamine), mescaline, psilocybin, nutmeg (myristical), Heavenly Blue morning glory seeds, marijuana (cannabis) and other hallucinogens all cause transitory toxic psychosis if taken in sufficient dosage for the particular individual. Psychotic effects may be related in part to underlying psychopathology and in part to a person's biochemical makeup. In susceptible individuals, a very little bit of marijuana can cause an acute paranoid psychotic reaction lasting two to three hours. Repeated L.S.D. use has resulted in a psychotic state requiring prolonged hospitalization.

All hallucinogens can present a clinical picture of depression, panic, paranoia, acute psychosis with hallucinations or confusion. If their use is suspected, but the exact drug is not known with certainty, caution must be exercised in treatment. A psychosis from D.M.T. can be greatly worsened by the use of Thorazine (chlorpromazine)!

It is true that the vast majority of marijuana users suffer no ill effects, but serious reactions must be kept in mind, as in pathologic intoxication on small doses of alcohol (see Chapter 11, "Drug Addiction and Alcoholism").

STIMULANT INTOXICATION

The effects of the amphetamines, Ritalin, cocaine and other stimulants range from excited alertness and euphoria to a "classical" paranoid psychosis with hallucinations and delusions of a persecutory nature. The amphetamines and cocaine are very highly addicting, generally believed to be more psychologically addicting than heroin, (addiction to stimulants also has a physiologic component differing from that of heroin). The severe mental symptoms appear after chronic usage and are absolutely indistinguishable from the functional psychoses except for the history of drug taking (when available).

There is no danger in treating these states with the major tranquilizers but the effect is not great until the use of the stimulants is stopped.

ALCOHOL INTOXICATION

This may take the form of acute or chronic syndromes induced by alcohol usage. Here too the effects vary according to the individual's underlying personality and possibly his biochemical makeup. The classical syndromes are defined as follows:

Simple Intoxication. A typical acute brain syndrome which is nonpsychotic. The picture is well known to all and ranges from talkativeness, expansiveness and euphoria through ataxia and clouding of consciousness to stupor. It may be confused with acute sedative intoxication (see p. 142) and may, of course, coexist with any psychiatric symptomatology. Because it is usually short lived, it presents no special problem to the nurse, except one of management.

Pathologic Intoxication. A syndrome which results from drinking small quantities of alcohol (in the susceptible individual). It is characterized by severe disorientation, violent or destructive behavior and amnesia. Susceptible persons in this case often have some degree of brain damage which should be investigated.

Delirium Tremens (D.T.s). Generally thought to be an abstinence syndrome in heavy drinkers in which metabolic and nutritional factors may play a part. Early signs are restlessness and irritability, progressing to confusion, disorientation and terrifying hallucinations (e.g., pink elephants). Convulsions may occur. Treatment should be in a hospital. It would be very unusual not to know the cause of the hallucinations (the patient readily states he needs a drink). Besides, their content and form is characteristic. *As many as two or three out of five cases may die if untreated.*

Korsakoff's Psychosis. May appear alone or in combination with other alcoholic syndromes. It may also be caused by various other poisons and toxins. Diagnosis is suggested by the finding of *confabulation* in which memory gaps are filled by falsehoods, not recognized by the patient as such.

Alcoholic Paranoid State. A syndrome developing in chronic alcoholism characterized by jealousy and delusions of infidelity. With or without the history of alcoholism it is quite difficult to distinguish from a paranoid psychosis. (See also amphetamine intoxication.)

Alcoholic Hallucinosis. A syndrome with a clear sensorium (c.f., all other alcoholic syndromes) in which the patient experiences terrifying auditory hallucinations of an accusing or threatening nature. This must also be distinguished from the functional paranoid states.

Alcoholic Deterioration. The "'burned out" alcoholic. Rarely a diagnostic problem. These sad people show personality and intellectual deterioration from years of drinking. They often have neurologic signs such as tremor, weakness and dysarthria.

Trauma

Following head injuries there may be irritability, decreased ambition and tolerance to stress, irresponsibility, lability of affect, poor concentration and memory defects, all of which represent the organic brain syndrome secondary to loss of brain tissue. A Korsakoff-like syndrome (with confabulation) may occur. Also, due to the psychologic reaction to the injury (especially where the functioning of the mind was highly valued by the patient), symptoms of anxiety, depression and withdrawal may occur. There is rarely any confusion regarding diagnosis following trauma if the history of injury is known.

Intracranial Neoplasm

Personality changes are often the first signs of brain tumor and usually recognized in retrospect. Typical psychotic symptoms may accompany frontal and temporal lobe tumors. The presence of visual or olfactory hallucinations should make one begin to consider the possibility of organicity, and in the presence of the other indicators of organic brain syndrome (see p. 140) should lead to further investigation. Like syphilis, some cases of slowgrowing tumors in relatively silent areas of the brain (producing no neurologic symptoms) have resulted in psychologic "treatment" for years, the diagnosis being made at autopsy. However, some of the procedures used to diagnose brain tumor are both dangerous in themselves and expensive, and should not be used unless definite indications are present.

Just as there is a "feel" for the natural history of functional emotional illness, the nurse specializing in neurology also develops a "feel" for the natural history of organic brain disease, and can detect subtle changes indicative of organicity that often go unnoticed by a psychiatric nurse.

It would be ideal if a nurse-consultant in neurology could spend time in the mental health center on a regular basis in exchange for a psychiatric nurse in the neurology clinic. A similar exchange between psychiatry and internal medicine would be equally fruitful.

Cerebral Arteriosclerosis

Confusion, memory loss, and behavioral changes of all types occur intermittently but progressively in many elderly patients and may coexist with senility. Barbiturates should be used cautiously, if at all, because they frequently cause delirium in these patients. This should be remembered because nighttime excitement often occurs, and could lead the unwary doctor or nurse into considering a barbiturate for its sedative effect. Also, any drug with hypotension as a side effect may precipitate hypoperfusion of cerebral vessels, causing stroke. Cerebral arteriosclerotic disease is seen more frequently now that more and more services are being extended by centers to the elderly.

Nutritional, Metabolic and Endocrine Disorders

These disorders would pose no special problem to the community nurse if all patients received a complete medical workup, including laboratory studies, upon beginning treatment at a mental health center. Federal funding for mental health, however, does not provide for this sort of screening, and the nurse, particularly in a rural area, or in a center not affiliated with a general hospital, will often have to decide whether or not medical studies are indicated. In most cases the physical signs and symptoms themselves are sufficient to bring attention to the illness, but often the "emotional disorder" is the first indication of a disease process.

Awareness and alertness diminish, and memory and orientation are affected, as the earliest and most subtle signs of metabolic brain disease. The nurse should consider metabolic disorder in every patient whose thinking, behavior, or state of consciousness has recently become disturbed.

HYPERTHYROIDISM (Thyrotoxicosis)

The patient is nervous, weak, restless and overactive with weight loss, sweating and tremor. This condition can be confused with anxiety states and manic disorders. Also, the presence of increased appetite, sensitivity to heat, palpitation, exophthalmos, or stool frequency should bring this disease to mind. The diagnosis is made by laboratory studies.

HYPOTHYROIDISM (Myxedema)

Early fatigue, sleepiness and constipation appear as in depression. When the course of this disease is prolonged or severe, hallucinations, disorientation, paranoid thinking and even suicide attempts are known. Symptoms and signs that help in differentiation are: brittle and coarse hair, sparse lateral eyebrow hair, thickened dry skin, diminished hearing and puffy or watery eyes.

UREMIA

Early symptoms in slowly progressive renal disease are lassitude and fatigue. If the polyuria goes unnoticed, depression may be diagnosed mistakenly. Restlessness may develop later, and physical symptoms including headache, nausea, vomiting, diarrhea, pruritus, hiccough and chest pain may also appear, helping to make the diagnosis. In *late renal failure* toxic psychosis with confusion, hallucinations and delusions sometimes occur with intervals of insight. These patients are, and appear to be, physically very sick.

HYPOGLYCEMIA

This condition may produce apathy, disorientation, confusion and weakness. Hunger is usually present and the patient should be questioned about using insulin or alcohol. (*All* patients should be asked these questions regardless of the presence of symptoms.) It must be remembered that insulin is occasionally used for suicidal (or homicidal) purposes.

HYPERGLYCEMIA

Itching, hunger, weakness and weight loss are seen along with polyuria and thirst. Chronic hyperglycemia can appear as depression early in the course of the illness, especially as diabetes often develops over many years. Hyperglycemia can be produced by diuretics (often taken by neurotic women for real or imagined obesity) and by lithium salts in some patients (used in the treatment of cyclothymic illness).

PORPHYRIA

This illness may present with a long history of nervousness, emotional instability and a variety of functional disturbances. Most striking, when they occur, are personality changes, psychoses, confusional states and hysterical symptoms. An acute attack is accompanied by colicky abdominal pain, severe vomiting, persistent constipation and occasional diarrhea. Precipitating the acute attack may be barbiturates, birth control pills, menses, or pregnancy and delivery.

HEPATIC ENCEPHALOPATHY

Personality changes here may include depression or euphoria, irritability, anxiety, paranoia and loss of concern for persons or property. There may be disturbances of consciousness, memory and concentration. (See p. 144, "alcoholism".)

PELLAGRA (niacin deficiency) and
BERIBERI (thiamine (B_1) deficiency)

A syndrome marks the onset of both deficiencies, characterized by depression, apathy, apprehension and fear, with anorexia, irritability and memory difficulties.

In pellagra, mania and delirium or frank paranoia is often seen, with delusions and hallucinations.

Most vitamin deficiencies are multiple when the general nutrition is poor. However pellagra is seen in areas where the diet consists of a great deal of corn and beriberi where there is liver disease, most commonly from alcoholism.

PERNICIOUS ANEMIA (B_{12} deficiency)

Cerebral involvement may cause euphoria, clouding of consciousness and psychotic behavior. The smooth red tongue and gastrointestinal symptoms aid in differentiating this disease from other organic and functional conditions.

Senile and Presenile Dementias

In these condtions there is usually a progressive intensification of the patient's former personality traits and characteristic behaviors. Social isolation and physical illness may intensify the process. The presenile dementias may begin in the forties and progress insidiously. They are often misdiagnosed initially and presently have no specific treatment. They should be thought of when other signs of organic brain syndrome appear or the patient fails to respond to ordinary treatments.

Degenerative Disease of the Central Nervous System

HUNTINGTON'S CHOREA

May appear in the teens but usually does not appear until age 30. This inherited disorder often appears as an emotional illness before the distinctive neurologic signs of choreo-athetosis, ataxia and speech disturbance show themselves.

MULTIPLE SCLEROSIS

Characterized by exacerbations and remissions of great variability. Mental symptoms include emotional lability, euphoria, depression and irritability. Usually the neurologic signs and symptoms are characteristic along with the remitting history.

CONCLUSION

All of the above are listed and briefly described to alert the nurse and to remind her that her medical background is indispensable to her role in community mental health. Perhaps the mystique of "becoming a psychotherapist" is fading somewhat in nursing and medical schools, but it is still a powerful motivation for certain students. Being a psychotherapist in no way diminishes the need to acquire and to maintain general nursing skills. The nurse's unique position, like the doctor's, in a situation where all other professionals are without medical training, should call forth all of her nursing experience and knowledge and then some.

FURTHER READING

Detre, Thomas P. and Jarecki, Henry G. Modern Psychiatric Treatment. Philadelphia: J. B. Lippincott, 1971. pp. 396-448.

11

Drug Addiction and Alcoholism

INTRODUCTION

Depending on how they are defined, these disorders are forms of mental illness, or physiochemical diseases, or social ills. They are "treated" more by laymen than by mental health professionals in such organizations as Synanon and Alcoholics Anonymous. The physical aspects of withdrawal are seen as medical problems by many psychiatrists, and as psychiatric problems by many internists. Everyone wants the addictive diseases treated, just so long as it is done by somebody else. The reason is that no one knows how to treat these diseases and, indeed, there may well be no single treatment that can ever do the job.

NO SINGLE ADDICTIONS

To begin with, there are no single addictions known. The man who says he is only addicted to heroin is also addicted to the whole process of acquiring and administering the heroin to himself. He is addicted to the life style he has developed, to the summarized portion of life that he relates to as if it were all of life and all of the world. He does it because it is more comfortable to do than not to do—at least initially. People inject water, mayonnaise and any conceivable injectable substance when they cannot get a drug. They like to see the blood come back into the syringe or eyedropper. They like to see their vein stand up.

Drugs themselves are very frequently taken alternately or in combination, such as "ups" and "downs." The point made here is that even with seemingly single-drug addiction there are many other addictive elements in the person's life and behavior that support the drug addiction and maintain it.

DRUGS AND PREDICTABILITY

A person taking drugs gets addicted to the predictability they offer. In life, happy is chancy, high is certain. Compared to masturbation, sex with another person is complicated, involved, unpredictable and difficult to maintain control over. With another, sex is dependent in part on the partner's moods, interest and (even messier) attraction to you at the time. Masturbation is neat, clean, private, utterly predictable and dependent upon no one else. So with drug taking. It is easy to get addicted to certainty, especially when uncertainty is frightening.

A person who says "I only use heroin" is today certain of his supply. When the supply is in question he will use speed or cocaine or methadone almost without exception.

LIFE STYLE AND MYTHOLOGY

The life style of drug taking has a strong appeal. It is often like playing the lead role in a cops-and-robbers movie. It is like belonging to a secret organization with its own language and with an esoteric body of knowledge that the public does not know. There are inside jokes, numerous stories to tell and to listen to about drugs, inside heroes and villains to praise and condemn. While Middle America is boring itself to death in suburbia with its cocktail parties and barbecue pits and club meetings, the drug takers are doing what they want, feeling what they want and controlling their own destiny when and how they want. While Middle America gets outraged at the spread of drug taking, many users confidently tell each other that this is because Middle America secretly wants to get high too, but it is afraid. Just as homosexuals often see all people as "latent" or potentially homosexual, drug users see all people as "latent junkies" (see p. 67.) If people could just throw over those great social evils—the Protestant ethic and the work ethic—then they would be free. Free to take drugs and do whatever they wanted to do.

Drug takers have their own history, as long and venerable as the history of the world. There were poets, writers, philosophers, kings who were addicted to drugs or alcohol. Freud in his enthusiasm for cocaine got a goodly portion of the royalty of Europe hung up on it. Winston Churchill drank a bottle of brandy a day. The southwest American Indians are permitted by the government to use Peyote (mescaline) in their religious ceremonies. East Indians have been into hashish for centuries. Grass is ubiquitous on the campuses of America.

Consider the following arguments. Much of the degradation of drug taking is due to the criminal aspects of it and this is solely due to society having made it a crime. If it were legal to buy heroin cheaply and to use it, then those who wanted it would not have to steal to get the money for it. If someone wants to put something in his vein, whose business is it anyway? Isn't it his vein? Are the people who work and pay taxes so angry at their position they must insist that everyone work and pay taxes? If so, they are really stupid. By making drug taking a crime they have cost themselves an incredible amount of money. And so on.

Did you follow the above arguments? Did you find them point by point reasonable, but in their entirety something that made you uneasy? Did you want to disagree with this "logical" mythology but not quite know where to begin? This argument and many like it were presented by a drug user over several years of psychotherapy with a skillful therapist. The drug user won the argument. He is dead.

THE NURSE'S POSITION

The fledgling therapist approaching the drug taker with a clear but naive view of drugs as evil, and with good, solid middle class values, will find herself quickly on the defensive and often unable to justify her values. It is not uncommon for the nurse to encounter patients who refuse treatment while admitting that they know they need it or that they know at least it is "the best thing" for them. Under ordinary circumstances, however, the nurse rarely encounters patients who question the entire therapeutic process and societal standards in general while presenting very compelling arguments supporting their own position. What nurse has not asked herself if the hassles of nursing school are worth it? Who has not wondered if being law abiding really pays off? Who has not considered the "helping professions" as having a bit too much masochism and self-sacrifice about them to be "really healthy" pursuits? This very questioning and openness that makes for the difference between a sensitive, really effective nurse and a reliable, ordinary nurse can lead the best students into wanting to know what makes junkies tick and into wanting to help them. This knowledge and these skills can be gotten, but not easily. It takes a lot of experience and soul-searching to reach the maturity to know who you really are, what you believe in and why, and still remain open and loving. It also takes time. It has been estimated that ten years' experience after professional school is needed for a person to develop the degree of wisdom required to handle herself with ease and grace with hard-core addicts.

Add to this the particular vulnerability of nurses and doctors to become addicted themselves and it becomes abundantly clear why most health professionals shy away from the entire addiction problem as being untreatable, and are quite content to leave the matter in the hands of groups of ex-addicts and nondrinking alcoholics.

Given these conditions, what role can the community mental health nurse fill? What is her area of competence? When should her personal safety commend her to inaction lest her enthusiasm and curiosity lead her into deceptively dangerous areas?

Each nurse and each mental health center must make these determinations and periodically rethink them as situations change.

WHO TO TREAT AND WHERE

When a drug-taking* patient has a demonstrable mental illness, regardless of the cause, he is a legitimate candidate for mental health center treatment. He may be schizophrenic or depressed, have an amphetamine psychosis or Korsakoff's syndrome. The treatment of these disorders in a drug-taker is not unlike their treatment in anyone else with the exception of certain safeguards to protect other people and their property.

When drug taking (and alcoholism) is defined as "mental illness" in and of itself by Federal regulations (as it is), then community mental health centers have an obligation to see that these patients receive treatment, even when ordinary mental illness cannot be demonstrated. It is not required, however, that they be mixed in with the other patients or even treated at the mental health facility itself. The centers may, and often do, provide consultative services to outside drug and alcohol units, and may have contractual arrangements with them so that mental health funds can flow through the center to the agency providing care.

However, when such arrangements have not been made, the nurse may find herself in the position of being asked to provide individual or group therapy to drug takers or alcoholics who do not have demonstrable mental illness. This situation will be discussed here with primary emphasis on attitudes and approaches that afford maximum safety to the nurse.

THERAPY OF THE ADDICT WITHOUT MENTAL DISORDER

Assessing The Conflict

Mental health professionals are being called upon more and more to treat addiction with the methods which have been developed to treat the psychotic and neurotic disorders. In those addicted persons who show no sign of these major or minor mental illnesses it is often necessary to modify therapy considerably and indeed to devise new ways of approaching the problem.

In a full-blown addictive disorder there are several factors which support and perpetuate the addiction. These are: (1) The addictive properties of the chemical(s) used. (2) The fear of withdrawal phenomena. (3) Social support by the drug-using community. (4) Fear of survival in the "straight world" (competition, sex, work, etc.). (5) Attraction to the comfort and simplicity of the addiction. (6) The pull of the obsessive-compulsive ritual of the addiction. (7) The lack of preparation for "straight" life (job skills, schooling, etc.).

Any two of these are sufficient to support an addiction.

On the other side, there are certain factors which might bring an addicted person in for help. These include: (1) Encounters with the law, or fear of same. (2) Deteriorating physical health or fear of such.

*Refers to alcoholics also, unless they are specifically excluded.

(3) Pressure from family and/or friends. (4) Disgust or disenchantment with the addiction. (5) Desire to cut back the habit for financial reasons. (6) Love.

Once the determination of addiction without mental illness has been made, the nurse should assess the factors supporting the addiction and weigh them against the factors that bring the patient in for help. This way some idea may be gotten about how deeply the patient is involved in the addictive process and how much motivation there is to consider change. All these factors do not carry equal weight, by any means. For example, an arrest, a suspended sentence and a very strict probationary period are often highly motivating and often life-saving. Also, in certain persons, being loved in the depths of addiction is a powerful stimulus to change.

Drug History

The next question has to do with whether the patient is currently using drugs or has quit, and for how long. Nothing can be done with someone who is drunk or nodding from heroin. He should be sent home in the company of some reliable person and told to return when he is not intoxicated.

A drug history can be taken from a nonintoxicated user but it should be considered a poetic offering rather than a factual report. Patients wanting methadone or barbiturates will invariably inflate their reported use by a factor of two in order to allow for the therapist's disbelief and still be given enough not to hurt. Although the decision to maintain a person on or withdraw him from drugs is a medical one, a separate history by the nurse is always valuable. Patients often forget their story in the retelling and it is well to check out the several versions.

Users and Nonusers

If the patient is presently "sober" and not a candidate for drug substitution of any kind, but is still "using," should therapeutic efforts proceed? There is divided opinion on this. Many feel that the patient should be entirely off drugs for a period of time before any treatment of the addiction can be considered. This is a valid position. Others prefer to be more lenient, saying that many drug users cannot begin to stop until they have received some encouragement and help. This is also true. However, it seems most reasonable to keep the nonusers and users separated so that the different approaches used on these groups can be more specifically applied.

USERS

Users should be required to refrain from drugs on the days they come to the center, and this minimum extended as they develop more strength. When first seeing a drug user the therapist must make it absolutely clear that she will never give him drugs or money (even for a telephone call)—and stick to it. She must keep any medicine, her pocketbook, valuables and prescription blanks locked up at all times, and inform other workers in the center to do the same. All typewriters, adding machines, radios, phonographs and similar valuable equipment must be kept in locked rooms and preferably also bolted down by the maintenance department so that they cannot be removed. The therapist must inform the patient that she doesn't trust him by virtue of her knowledge and experience with drug takers, even though she would like to, and that she looks forward to the day when she can.° She must tell the patient that little can be done until he quits but that she can listen to his plans to quit and to his plans for the future. She can encourage him to socialize with people out of the drug culture, to get an easy job, to think about school, or whatever. The nurse must keep firmly in mind that there is nothing that she can do directly to stop the patient from using drugs. She must remember that he may die or go to prison, or succumb to bacterial endocarditis, and there is nothing she can do about that. These possibilities should also be told to the patient (if only to let the patient know that *she* knows). The nurse must be non-judgmental, and neither preach nor exhort. She may comment that drug taking seems stupid to her and wonder when the patient last experimented with not using, and how it went. She may outline the help that the center can offer to the user when he is drug-free. Her approach must be a "softsell" while toughly protective of herself. What she offers is kindness, realistic concern, and a consistent placing of the responsibility for quitting where it can only be—with the patient.

Probation. If the patient is in treatment through a probation department the nurse must remind the patient of the conditions of the probation and her duty (or the center's duty) to report any deviance. Since psychiatric probation requires that the patient be drug-free, the patient may be reluctant to report occasional drug taking or, on the other hand, may want to enlist the nurse as an ally in his back-sliding. If the therapist is to do the reporting, she should get to know the probation officer, at least by telephone, and get some sense of how much leeway he will permit. It is rare for an addicted person to stop cold and never to try drugs again. If the return to drugs is sporadic, and efforts to get a life together are genuine, most probation officers will be understanding—to a point. The nurse should take great care not to become the patient's ally against his probation officer, or be worked into the position where she is seen as a "rat." This should be clearly set forth in the initial interview.

Add to all of these cautions the problems that a bright, manipulative, verbal patient can generate, and the nurse or physician may wisely decide that such "therapy" is beyond her scope.

°Patients will complain about this attitude. "You're my therapist—at least you should trust me. How can I get better if you don't believe in me?" Later, after stopping the use of drugs they will probably volunteer that your tough line was actually reassuring to them and that you were right because "no junkie can ever be trusted."

NONUSERS

There is pretty general agreement that nonusers should be handled in a group therapy situation. All of the considerations already stated regarding users also apply here. The principles of "getting a life together" (see Chapter 5, Psychotherapy") are as valid for nonusing drug takers as for recovering mentally ill patients.

Prognosis. A very important prognostic consideration is how much of a life the patient had together before addiction began. The earlier the addiction started, the lower the educational level, the shorter the job record—the poorer the prognosis. A man who stops drugs at age 25 after ten years of use may have to face high school and/or the acquisition of job skills for the first time, and that is not easy.

Several ex-addicts in a group or an entire group of them pose certain problems. The tendency to reminisce and talk about the old days and "how many bags-a-day habit I had" is strong. Very mature ex-addicts trained in psychotherapy are quite valuable as therapists or co-therapists and can usually stop this "junkie" talk with dispatch. There is no magic in being an ex-addict, however, and it is certainly no substitute for training and experience in psychotherapy.

Drugs Change The Personality

Somewhere in all these struggles with a patient who is bent on his own destruction and seemingly knows it the nurse must ask herself, "Who am I talking to? What kind of a person is this who is so sure of his fear of life that he is totally absorbed in the business of killing himself off for five to ten hours at a stretch until it's done permanently? Do people really have the right to take their own lives?" This ethical question can be answered and defended in several ways. More and more people today are asserting that this is indeed a person's right. As long as the property or life of others is not harmed, it is entirely up to each individual to determine when and how he shall die or live, as the case may be. Courts have defended patients' rights to refuse all sorts of treatment, life-saving and otherwise, so long as the patient is competent to make these decisions. In general terms, a person is considered incompetent when his customary good judgment and reason are not available to him, for whatever cause. Legally this is determined by the court. In most cases such determinations are made where the patient has shown poor judgment and unreasonableness for a protracted period of time, as in senility. Incompetency may be general or for specific things. In chronic alcoholism, for example, where the patient is declared incompetent to drive a motor vehicle, he may be seen as competent to handle his affairs in other aspects of life.

Many drugs cause organic brain syndrome (see Chapter 10, "Medical Problems that Mimic or Complicate Emotional Disorders"). It is obvious to anyone that a person on L.S.D. who "decides" he should fly out of a 10th story window is not "competent" to make that decision at that time, without the necessity of a court hearing to determine it legally. Such a person has an acute organic brain syndrome, and is not "in his right mind." So with someone who is intoxicated with any substance. In a situation of *chronic* intoxication, each decision to take more drugs is made by a person whose brain functioning is impaired by the previous dose he took. To argue logically with such a person about whether he should or should not take more drugs or kill himself is as foolish as arguing with a person experiencing D.T.'s that there aren't bugs crawling over him. Both have an organic brain syndrome, one being more subtle than the other. The most reasonable treatment might well be to lock up and dry out all addicted persons and then to ask them what they want to do with their lives. This is not possible, however, and we must deal with the system as it is, for it is designed to protect the rights of most of the people. However, the dilemma of the therapist must be clearly seen, as should the importance of abstinence before meaningful therapy can take place.

THE ADDICTIVE LIFE STYLE

What about the addict's arguments presented in the beginning of the chapter? Is addiction a valid life style for some? What is a valid life style? Is being a soldier and killing people a valid life style?

The nurse need not answer these questions for the addict because he is not seeking answers. He is seeking to justify his behavior intellectually because he has become convinced that there is no changing it. The nurse must answer the questions for herself, however, because nothing is quite as reassuring as a person who knows what she is about, and nothing as unsettling as a person (therapist) who lacks confidence about the very basis on which her own life style is established.

WHAT IS A VALID LIFE STYLE?

As described in Chapter 5, "Psychotherapy," movement in the direction of maturity is healthy. A life style that promotes this is valid. The standard against which validity is judged is the person's own potential. Enough is known about human potential in general to make some rather clear statements about what a person can expect when moving towards his potential and how he will look to an observer.

A valid life style promotes growth and development at any age, has variety, encourages the taking of reasonable risks, provides for adaptability, utilizes most of a person's resources, allows for joy. The person with a valid life style can lose any element in it and not lose his life.

An invalid life style has limited options, restricts growth and development, is not readily adaptable to change, has few risks and many guaranteed outcomes (not all good ones), may permit a measure of happiness—but never joy.

Is addiction a valid life style? Never! Not whether it is an addiction to drugs, or alcohol, or sex, or work, or playing, or eating or any other manner of consuming activity. Can a "small addiction" (like smoking cigarettes) be part of a valid life style? Yes, but it doesn't add anything to the overall validity of such a life. It detracts from it.

Can a valid life style contain an element in it that is of questionable philosophic soundness? Yes. Take the example of the career soldier, married, with children, happy, with friends, able to enjoy sports and reading, taking extension courses in a favorite subject and progressing satisfactorily in his vocation. This has the characteristics of a valid life style, whether or not we believe in soldiering and war. If this man is adaptable enough to reconsider his vocational choice, and has enough other supports and involvements in life to allow him to do this, and to move on and change jobs if he so decides, his life style is valid. One's style refers to how one handles oneself, not what one does for a living or a hobby. The addicted person is not adaptable in this way, and is quite resistant to change.

HITTING BOTTOM

It is the experience of many workers in the area of drugs and alcohol that help is not possible until the patient has "hit bottom." This means that all the "factors that might bring a person in for help" (see p. 152), with the exception of love, are present. With drug takers this occurs earlier than with alcoholics and consists of the loss of all the elements in an ordinary life plus physical ill health. It usually means several arrests, some time in prison (especially for drug takers) and utter poverty.

After the discouragement and heartbreak of dealing with addicted persons over the years, it is understandable how this belief in the seeming necessity of utter degradation develops. It is apparently a necessary condition for treatment in certain patients, and is a view that serves to protect the feelings of the therapist. "John quit treatment but he'll be back. He hasn't bottomed out yet." We take exception to the universal application of this principle. There are enough addicts of all types who do not have to "bottom out" to warrant more optimism than this belief holds. If the therapist is cynically waiting for the bottom to appear, the patient will most likely be dead (especially with drug takers) before this occurs. If the patient has enough motivation to come for help, then a sense of urgency to secure that help for him is warranted. If he is still using chemicals, getting him dry is the first order of business and may best be done in a hospital or special residential treatment setting. If not, the possibility of prison should be considered if this can be arranged. The description given earlier of considerations in the individual treatment of the current user is to help with those cases where no satisfactory or acceptable alternative arrangement can be made.

If your brother were hooked on speed, to what extent would you explore different treatment possibilities before concluding that he can't be helped until he "bottoms out?"

THE SOCIABLE ADDICTIONS

There are a multitude of people in America with addictive disorders who remain hidden in the fabric of society because they never break the law or behave in a bizarre way. They may be addicted to introducing various chemicals and substances into their bodies or addicted to some behavior. Writers tend to reserve the term "addiction" for those habits involving chemicals which produce physical symptoms of withdrawal when their use is terminated. The term "habituation" generally refers to dependence on those chemicals which do not produce physical symptoms of withdrawal when stopped. The phrase "obsessive compulsive habit pattern" is used for those habitual, repetitive behaviors which the patient cannot easily stop.

In our experience, the motivation for all three is basically the same, and patients who begin to move in therapy almost always move around in the area of "addictive behavior" for quite some time before they move out of it. It is not at all unusual for a person to shift from one chemical to another, and then to cigarettes and alcohol, and then to sex and food and then to work in the course of treatment. Such persons will hold on as tenaciously to their behavior as they held on to their chemical. They see any interference as a threat to their existence, and will not permit it. Having seen someone change in this way convinces the observer that they are now "work junkies" instead of "heroin junkies." In no way do we mean to imply that this change is not good, desirable and healthy. It is all of these. But it is not basic change. The style is the same. However, because their new obsession is praised by society, productive and physically healthy, they will feel far better. Most will settle gladly for the improvement. Unless some catastrophe strikes, their new method of operation will probably stick, and serve them well. A few will insist on continuing to work in therapy until they have broken out of the addictive style altogether. These people achieve real freedom.

Approaching the addictive continuum from the other (socially acceptable) direction we find many who will never continue to the point of narcotic addiction, and hardly ever consider their life style as addictive, but it is. The obese are addicted to eating. Smokers are addicted to tobacco and smoking behaviors. There are to 16- to 18-hour-a-day hard-driving businessmen who "can't stop work." Anxious, trapped housewives may be addicted to minor tranquilizers and daytime television. There are "social drinkers" who "must" have their 5 p.m. martini and several more and who get very uncomfortable if they can't easily get it. There are sleep addicts who spend 10 hours in bed each night and 12 to 14 on weekend nights (with a nap when they can work it in).

What do these people have in common? They all feel they need to do what they are doing. They all feel (from time to time) that they should stop. They all try to stop and fail. They all develop ways of justifying to themselves and others that what they do is OK but they don't really believe it. They all derive some comfort from their activity and they all feel trapped by it.

There is much to be said for this view of addictive human behavior. It should blur somewhat the prejudicial distinction between the "evil, inhuman junkie" and the "model hard-working (over-working) citizen." After all, it really isn't possible for a human being to do something "inhuman," is it? Or to be a "model person"?

RECREATIONAL CHEMICALS

Men have used chemical substances for recreation (fun, relaxation, diversion, etc.) for all of recorded history. In all likelihood they will continue to do so for many more years. The question is asked "Why should people have to take something to feel good? Isn't it natural to feel good? Why can't they do it on their own?" It would seem reasonable, given the limitlessness of the human mind, that they *could* "do it on their own," but few do. When, however, an unbelievably minute speck of L.S.D. can create a mental state that hardly anyone achieves after a lifetime of yoga and meditation, the attraction is undeniable. Dangerous as acid may be, it opens up possibilities for biochemical alteration of thoughts and moods that are staggering. Naturally occurring hallucinogens have been used for centuries in most parts of the world in nonaddictive ways.

The day is fast approaching when Aldous Huxley's fictional "soma" will be a reality—a universal "happy pill."

Alcohol is certainly America's number one recreational chemical, and probably the world's It is used in nonaddictive ways by most people but there are no statistics to substantiate this belief.

Marijuana is so widely used today that laws prohibiting it are currently under review.

What is a sane and common-sense approach to this entire recreational chemical situation? If we believe in a glass of wine with dinner, we believe in recreational chemicals. What other drugs are as harmless in this dosage and for this purpose? Probably marijuana. What are too dangerous to consider? Any drugs that are physically addicting (the narcotics), that frequently cause psychosis in low dosage (the amphetamines and some hallucinogens), that produce automatic behavior and resultant "accidental overdosage" (the barbiturates), and those that produce convulsions and other "release phenomena" on cessation (most C.N.S. depressants).

The only problem with this logical construction is that there is one chemical that meets all these "too dangerous to consider" criteria. That chemical is ethyl alcohol.

When a person is using something occasionally that he has under control, that is not dangerous in the dosage used, to which he is not addicted and on which he is not dependent (he truly does not "need" it), and which gives him pleasure, then the mental health disciplines really have nothing to say about the matter. It is out of their area of concern and competence. Legal and religious groups may have something to say about it, and often do. We wish to opt for taking a public stand only on matters where we have some expertise.

THE METHADONE MYTH

Methadone (dolophine) is a synthetic narcotic that has certain useful properties. (1) It is effective orally. (2) Its duration of action is two to three times longer than that of heroin and other opiate narcotics, and so it can be used just once a day. (3) It can be substituted for other opiates and completely prevent physical withdrawal symptoms. (4) In high enough doses it produces a "narcotic blockade" action that prevents the user from getting "high" on other narcotics while on the methadone.

The bulk of early research on methadone was done in New York by Nyswander and Dole[1] who showed that heroin addicts could be switched to methadone orally once a day and, in the proper (maintenance) dose could be kept off of heroin and returned to gainful employment. The methadone satisfied their physical craving for an opiate substance, and effectively removed them from the criminal drug world where they had obtained their heroin, and from the criminal activities that they had engaged in to pay for their habit.

The researchers had not finished their work, had not yet obtained any long-range followup studies, but had concluded that methadone maintenance patients should concurrently receive some sort of psychotherapy, when the methadone issue was pulled from the medical to the political arena and made an issue of national concern. Methadone was called the "answer to the addiction problem" which obviously it is not, nor was ever intended to be. It has absolutely no application in the rehabilitation of pill takers, speed freaks, acid heads, cocaine users or alcoholics. Its sole use is with opiate narcotic users and has two applications there. First, for withdrawal, it is useful for helping someone to stop heroin usage without painful physical withdrawal symptoms. Used this way in decreasing doses for five days to two weeks it is quite helpful. This use should probably be restricted to a hospital setting where there is a drug-free environment so that the drug of abuse (heroin) is not available as an option to the patient. Second, for maintenance, it is useful in selected patients as a substitute, legal addiction which will permit them to function in a relatively normal fashion. The overwhelming problem here, by no means adequately researched as yet, is that these still-addicted patients have a strong tendency to take other drugs along with the methadone (see *No Single Addictions*, p. 149) such as cocaine and the amphetamines and C.N.S. depressants.

Nonetheless, Federal and state funds have been allocated to cities for establishment of methadone maintenance clinics as a solution to the "drug problem," and they have sprung up like mushrooms, often without the intensive psychotherapy dimension recommended by the founders of the method. How long this situation will last and how effective methadone used in this way will prove to be remains to be seen. Many professionals are skeptical.

DANGEROUS DOCTORS

Most patients with emotional problems are seen and treated, not by psychiatrists or at mental health centers, but by family physicians, internists and dermatologists. The quality of care that the patients receive varies widely according to the training, skill, available time and native ability of these doctors. Some welcome the opportunity to treat "the whole patient" while others resent having to deal with "imaginary illnesses." Unfortunately a few appear to be willing to do anything to get the "neurotics" out of their offices. These men give amphetamines to stout people, C.N.S. depressants to insomniacs (no matter how mild) and minor tranquilizers to virtually anyone who is anxious. When the patients become dependent on these drugs or when more severe mental symptoms begin to appear, they show up in the psychiatrist's office or at the mental health center. The situation can usually be clarified by a careful and sensitive interview, but not always. The patients often like their "outside doctor," feel they "need" the medicine he has prescribed, and want to continue seeing him and taking the drugs while the mental health center treats their depression or whatever symptom brings them in. This is a very difficult and touchy business. A patient whose depression has been deepened, if not actually caused, by high doses of minor tranquilizers or C.N.S. depressants must be convinced of the importance of discontinuing his medicine before starting on an antidepressant or whatever psychotropic medication is appropriate.

Further, such patients have become conditioned to feeling no anxiety and having no sleep problems, and it is sometimes not possible to wean them away from the "prescribed medicine" on which they are dependent and to have them experience a bit of discomfort in the course of getting well.

The long-range solution, of course, is one of consultation and education with the psychiatric association, the county medical society and the community mental health center all working together. The handling of the individual patient, however, will call upon all of the diplomacy, maturity and inventiveness that the nurse can muster.

ALCOHOLISM

Social Pressure

The natural history of alcoholism differs in certain respects from that of other chemical addictions because the nonaddictive use of alcohol is permitted by law and supported and encouraged by the dominant society. In America it is our legal chemical of recreation and celebration, and is served at political functions and religious ceremonies. It is a central nervous system depressant.

In order to appreciate the strong social pressures to drink, every drinking therapist and student should take a three-month vacation from alcohol every two years while continuing ordinary life. Go to clubs, cocktail parties, dances and whatever else you enjoy, only drink club soda or ginger ale instead of wine, beer or whiskey. Notice the dismay of hosts and hostesses and friends as if something were wrong with them because you will not drink with them, or something wrong with you because you are no longer being "regular." Simply reply to their wonderment by saying "no thanks, I don't want to drink." Notice the pressure to "confess" that it is on "doctor's orders," or because you have a headache, or want to lose weight. Not drinking is strange and requires explanation. Not drinking is antisocial. Alcohol causes more highway deaths each year in America than all other chemicals put together.

Among young people, marijuana has replaced alcohol to a large extent, and enjoys the same social (but not legal) sanctions. If this is your chemical choice, stop smoking grass altogether for three months and hold out against the social pressure. Either way, it is an invaluable experience and should be considered as elective laboratory work in your study of the social forces in addiction. The argument—"I understand about social pressure. I'm not going to quit anything for three months like that. I could quit but I don't want to."—is not acceptable.°

Progression

There is no clear distinction at first between the behavior of the recreational (social) drinker and the addicted (problem) drinker. The difference involves the amount of compulsion to drink; this is rarely

---

°Because of the extraordinarily high addiction rate among medical personnel, we recommend a self-imposed three-month vacation from nonprescribed chemicals every two years throughout the nurse's professional life. Any difficulty in maintaining this schedule should alert her to seek help at once. The point being made here is that social pressures contribute to alcoholism. This is, of course, only part of the story. (See *Emotional and Physical Factors.*)

visible at first to either the observer or to the drinker. It is considered ordinary in some circles to have a drink with a business lunch and a 5 o'clock cocktail. What's wrong with a Bloody Mary or a Screwdriver with breakfast if you are at a convention and somebody else is picking up the tab?

Alcoholics Anonymous publishes a list of indicators that point to problem drinking, and one of their most valuable precepts is based on the compulsive element. "If you have to drink—don't!" It is not possible to tell, however, whether you just "want" a drink or actually "need" a drink if, each time you have the urge, you take the drink. If a person has not had an alcohol-free day for a long time, he may have little perception of how strong his compulsion to drink is. The housewife who has a drink after the children get off to school may feel she "deserves" it, and it is perfectly reasonable and "normal." When she gets to the point where she can't wait for them to leave and sneaks a little vodka into her orange juice at breakfast, she has a problem. So does the businessman who keeps a flask in his desk. So does the patient who brings a bottle into the hospital with him. When anyone "sneaks" a drink, he is trying to avoid criticism. "Other people wouldn't understand." The truth is that other people *would* understand quite clearly that the drinker is no longer drinking for recreation, but out of addiction, and if they had any feelings for the drinker they would tell him so and he would then be quite uncomfortable.

Further progression of the addiction involves deterioration in interpersonal relationships, job performance, mental clarity, emotional stability and physical health. Because it is legal to drink, and to purchase and possess alcohol, and because society sanctions drinking, a person who becomes addicted to alcohol often goes for years before he is recognized as such. It is characteristic of the alcohol addict (alcoholic) who has tried to quit many times with varying degrees of success but has always returned to drink, to know that he should not drink or at least believe that he should control his drinking, to feel guilty about the deprivation his drinking has caused his family, and still not to consider himself a "true alcoholic." The word "alcoholic" conjures up the image of the skid row bum, the derelict, the panhandler, the down-and-outer. In fact, however, only a very small percentage of alcohol addicts fit this image. To avoid the argument the word "alcoholic" should never be used with patients, unless they so identify themselves. Rather, speak of "problem drinking," or "compulsive drinking," or "secret drinking," or "alcohol addiction."

Taking The Drinking History

It is essential in every patient that the initial interviewer (the nurse or whoever) take a very careful and detailed history of drinking habits (See p. 13 *Drug and Alcohol History*). The questioning should be pointed and exhaustive. It must be remembered that alcohol addiction can coexist with any mental disorder, can make many disorders worse, and can occur in the absence of mental disorder altogether.

The Treatment of Alcohol Addiction

The treatment of alcohol addiction consists of the patient's recognizing his situation and stopping drinking completely—for life.

Treatment Aids

Various aids are used to assist the alcoholic in achieving and maintaining total sobriety, but they all require his cooperation and effort. There is no coercive treatment available.

PSYCHOTHERAPEUTIC TREATMENT

This treatment aid begins with a one-to-one relationship in which the patient can become dependent on and receive support from the therapist. Gradually the family is involved and the patient started in group therapy with other alcoholics. Finally, A.A. meetings can be used by the patient as he gains strength.

DISULFIRAM (ANTABUSE) TREATMENT

This drug interferes with the enzymatic breakdown of alcohol causing, when 15 to 60 cc of alcohol are taken, an acute acetaldehyde intoxication consisting of flushing, bloodshot eyes, headache, nausea and vomiting, palpitations and tachycardia, dyspnea, hyperventilation, sleepiness and hypotension. This reaction occurs within one and one-half hours of alcohol intake in the patient who has been maintained on Antabuse for two weeks or more.

The therapeutic rationale rests on the fear of responding to the impulse to drink, carrying the patient over time after time until the impulse can be handled without the help of Antabuse. The problem is that patients can discontinue Antabuse for several days and then drink.

The nurse should warn the patient on Antabuse to avoid *any* form of ethyl alcohol, including medicines with an alcohol base, alcohol rubs, foods and sauces prepared with alcohol and the breathing of alcohol fumes, as from shellac.

Average maintenance dose of Antabuse is 250 mg/day and the patient is given a test dose of alcohol to demonstrate its effect early in the treatment.

NEGATIVE CONDITIONING (AVERSION THERAPY)

Alcohol is given along with a nauseant such as apomorphine (2-8 mg) and repeated at regular intervals. The patient comes to associate the two and eventually gets sick just thinking about alcohol.

L.S.D.

L.S.D. has been used and reported to be successful in the treatment of some alcoholics. The process is lengthy and impractical but may open the door to other chemicals that facilitate insight.

REFERENCES

1. Dole, V.P. and Nyswander, M.E. "Rehabilitation of heroin addicts after blockade with methadone." *New York J. Med.*, 66:2011–2017, 1966.

FURTHER READING

Detre, Thomas P. and Jarecki, Henry G. Modern Psychiatric Treatment. Philadelphia: J.B. Lippincott, 1971; pp. 277-327.
Glasscote, Raymond M. et al. The Treatment of Alcoholism: A Study of Programs and Problems. Washington, D.C.: The Joint Information Service, 1967; pp. 1-31.

12

The Older Adult

INTRODUCTION

There is a tendency in America, more than in most countries, to value youth and to ignore the aging. This unnecessary emphasis on the first one third of the life span affects the patients we treat as well as ourselves. In this chapter we present a view of the aging process other than the prevailing one and urge the nurse to rethink her own position as she reads it.

Almost all the so-called problems of the elderly stem directly or indirectly from the obsolescence we build into the maturing and aging process, in much the same way as we do with the things we make. An automobile built in 1910 was made to last its owner for 20 to 30 years, was easy to repair at home and carried with it a tool kit and instruction manual so that repairs and adjustments could be made. An automobile built in the 1970's is made to last its owner for only two to three years, is difficult to repair at home and few people can make the necessary adjustments to keep it operating. This is primarily an American phenomenon and is much less true with foreign cars. The reasons for this business trend are easy to understand. By building obsolesence into cars, people will not worry about repairing them and keeping them up but will trade them in every few years. In this way they will always have a relatively new car with the latest equipment and be in fashion, and the auto manufacturers will always be busy. We are in the midst of the biggest "throw-away society" of all time.

We will not argue here as to our views on this attitude toward *things*. We do take vigorous exception to this attitude being applied to *people*. Human beings are built to last for 80 to 90 years with proper adjustments and repairs and as individuals there is no way for us to make a trade on a new model every 20 to 30 years. Nor would we want to. If society is viewed as the active agent, if society owns the cars (us), it can very easily trade us in for newer models, and does.

Thus, the throw-away society with built-in obsolescence has created a growing population of "useless," "outdated" people at the same time as it has created better and better methods and repair shops (medical technology and hospitals) to keep them going. It is the duty of the mental health profession to keep them sane. (But not productive. Productivity would mess up the social system.)

Let us look at the whole situation from various points of view and attempt to come to a sensible, workable position from which to operate with regard to our elderly patients, our present selves and our aging selves.

PRACTICAL CONSIDERATIONS

As people get older they tend to slow up. It takes them more time to get about, to express themselves and to make decisions. The mental health worker used to zipping along with younger patients usually feels frustrated and bogged down when dealing with the older adult. "It takes them so long to say what they mean." "I have to repeat directions over and over." "They keep asking the same questions. I get bored answering. I don't think they listen to me." This impatient reaction worries the elderly person, confuses him and slows things down even more. Old people know that you are busy and have a lot on your mind. They will understand if you have only a few minutes for them from time to time, so long as you spend more time when you have it. The older person's needs for physical health care, for financial help, for practical help with transportation, meals, and housing should be carefully and thoughtfully listened to and acted upon. The nurse who visits an aged person in his home will do well to take his blood pressure every week or two, to get up on a chair and replace the lightbulb in the ceiling fixture when it burns out, to have a cup of tea with him, to hang a picture when it falls down, to go over his diet with him and to write things down that he should remember. The 15 to 20 minutes that these take will more than pay off in the long run. Is this sort of thing mental health care? Yes, and of the highest order. It is primary prevention. In most areas of community mental health care, primary prevention is talked about but is too difficult to pin down to be truly workable. With the elderly, it is easy to do and works beautifully.

In this discussion we do not mean to imply that the nurse should be a housekeeper or baby sitter or "handyman." We do mean that she should be a human being and do the little things she can do without getting "hung up" in a formal definition of her "role." These things are highly symbolic to an older person and convey to him in clear and concrete terms that the nurse is interested in the whole person and in the quality of his life. They show that she is responsive to all of the person's needs, and that she cares.

In a comprehensive center, one functional element is devoted to services to the older adult. The staff of this element is geared to dealing with older persons and is aware of community resources that can be utilized to support and to sustain the aged. A day hospital facility available to or specializing in the elderly can be of great help when transient emotional difficulties arise. A socialization center (often located in a neighborhood church or community center) affords a meeting place for older people and need not be staffed by mental health personnel. However, its value is greatly increased if the mental health center has a liaison person there to explain the mental health services that are available, and to accept referrals on the spot.

Every effort should be made to keep the elderly out of institutions. The effect of institutionalization on the elderly is almost always devastating. However, in many a family's and young professional's mind, institutionalization is considered "inevitable sooner or later" and the prospect brings mixed feelings to all.

FACTS AND FANTASIES CONCERNING THE AGED

"The great majority of aged persons never display symptoms of senility. They show few or no signs of memory defect or other evidence of intellectual deterioration."[1] This fact comes as a shock to most health workers who have received an unbalanced view of the elderly in their training and experience. Our impressions represent the public mythology on aging in addition to our knowledge about the elderly with physical and mental disorders whom we have seen in hospitals, nursing homes and psychiatric facilities.

Of the 20 million persons in the United States today who are age 65 and older, less than one million are in institutions and three million live in the community with moderate to severe psychiatric impairment. This leaves 16 million elderly who are making some kind of successful adaptation to aging.

In general, the older adults who can be considered as successfully adjusted to their circumstances fall into one of three groups.

(1) The *mature* type, "with a constructive, active and involved approach to life."[2] "These people accept the facts of aging, adjust well to losses, are realistic about their past and present lives, and face death with equanimity."[3]

(2) The *armored* type, with "well-developed defenses, often of an overcompensating kind."[4] These people "cling to middle-aged behavior patterns, deny aging, keep as busy as ever, and manage to get along very well."[5]

(3) The *rocking chair* type, with "tendencies to lean on others and to be relatively passive."[6] This group is growing as society becomes more leisure oriented, and includes "people who accept passivity, and sit and rock without feeling guilty about it."[7]

While passivity and denial are generally considered as undesirable forms of adjustment among younger persons, they are frequently acceptable and quite workable for the elderly.

A summary of common fictions regarding the elderly and the facts that are known are presented side-by-side in Table 12-1.

TABLE 12-1

SUBJECT	FICTION	FACT
Definition of "elderly"	Based on biological fact.	A matter of socioeconomic policy. Coincides with retirement age of 65.
Socialization	The elderly would rather be alone.	The elderly desire access to others and want social interaction.
Health	The elderly as a group are both physically and mentally disabled.	Most elderly are healthy.
Institutions	Most elderly are in some type of institution.	Only five percent of the two million elderly live in institutions.
Housing in community	Elderly in the community either live in "retirement colonies" or in the homes of their children.	"Most of today's elderly maintain their own households."[8]
Death	Death is more feared by the elderly, who are closer to it in time than are the young.	Death is much more feared by the young than by the elerly, who are more concerned about financial security.
Retirement villages	It is better for the elderly to live with others who share similar interests and age-related concerns.	It is best for the elderly to remain in the general community, to associate with youth and to remain contemporary.
Psychiatric interview	It is more difficult to interview the elderly because they are evasive and confused.	The elderly are far more candid and direct in an interview situation. They are generally beyond "playing games."
Senility	Most elderly become senile.	Four fifths of the elderly show no signs of senility at any time.
Intellectual skills	Like physical powers, intellect fades progressively with increasing age.	In many areas involving intellect, judgment, knowledge and creativity, the elderly actually excel over their more youthful counterparts.
Homogeneity	While young adults differ from one another greatly, the elderly are all pretty much the same.	"Groupings based on chronological age are much less homogeneous in the old than in the young."[9]
"Old age" as a cause of death	Most people, if they live long enough, die of simple "old age."	Very few people, if any, die of "old age." Death is almost always due to physical causes such as cardiovascular disease or infection.
Suicide	The suicide rate is greater among the young.	"The suicide rate in white men over the age of 75 is more than seven times that of young adults in their early twenties."[10]

TABLE 12–1—(cont.)		
SUBJECT	**FICTION**	**FACT**
Needs of the elderly	Most elderly want less and need less than younger persons.	"The needs of aged persons are much like those of younger persons—to enjoy friendship and social contacts, to be busy at work and leisure activities in keeping with one's capacities, and to be in reasonably good health."[11]
Psychiatric impairment in the elderly	Due mostly to the aging process itself and social withdrawal.	Due more to physical ill health, often correctable, than any other factor studied.
Sex	The elderly are unconcerned about sex.	A satisfying sex life is not unusual among older persons to age 80 plus.

MENTAL HEALTH PROBLEMS OF THE AGED

General

The same mental health problems affect the elderly as those of any age, and treatment is essentially the same. For a detailed discussion of the varieties of mental disorder and their treatment you should consult the appropriate sections of this book. The emphasis here is on the *difference* encountered in the elderly person from the point of view of etiology, types of disorders most commonly seen and prognosis. *In general, nutritional problems and physical ill health rank much higher as causative factors in mental disorder in the elderly than in persons of younger years.* Also, recovery from acute psychiatric symptomatology is more rapid and complete with proper treatment than is usually thought to be the case.

Older adults are especially subject to stresses that are related to acute and chronic illnesses, decreased physical capacity, problems surrounding bereavement, retirement, social isolation and financial deprivation. Another cause of psychologic stress in the older adult (often profound) is radical environmental change, such as moves within the community or from home to institution or within the institution. Specific mental health problems will be considered here with a brief statement regarding their particular relationship to the elderly.

Organic Brain Syndrome

As discussed in Chapter 10 "Medical Problems that Mimic or Complicate Emotional Disorders," organic brain syndrome is subdivided into two types, related to both duration and etiology. They are acute brain syndrome (such as from acute toxic conditions or infections) and chronic brain syndrome (such as from chronic infections or circulatory disorders). In the elderly, when the cause of an *acute syndrome* can be identified as due to a specific physical illness, the results of adequate treatment are often a complete reversal of the psychologic symptoms. When a *chronic brain syndrome* is present (usually due to senile brain disease or cerebral arteriosclerotic brain disease), there is much less likelihood of reversal of the impairment.

Functional (Psychogenic) Disorders

Surprisingly, neurotic, schizophrenic and depressive illnesses tend to lessen in severity with aging. On the other hand, an unfavorable environment can induce hypochondriacal and depressive symptoms in the elderly. Recovery from these is possible by reducing the environmental stress.

Physical Ill Health

Physical ill health seems related to mental illness in the elderly more than any other factor studied. Physical illnesses such as heart failure, malnutrition, stroke, high blood pressure, respiratory infections, cancer and neuritis (usually associated with chronic alcoholism) are frequently found in the older adult with mental disorder. Often these illnesses are multiple.

Special Problems

Under this heading we include alcoholism, drug dependence, suicide and nutritional problems associated with psychiatric symptoms in the elderly.

ALCOHOLISM
One does not usually think of alcoholism as being a problem related to aging. However, it has been estimated that 25 percent of the aged admitted to mental hospitals suffer from alcoholism to a significant degree. Of this group one fourth began drinking heavily *after age 60* due to the stresses associated with the problems of aging.

DRUG DEPENDENCE
Aging drug misusers? Yes. The elderly frequently become dependent on central nervous system depressants or tranquilizers, which are prescribed because they complain of insomnia and pain so often. Such complaints usually vanish when appropriate assistance and thoughtful attention are given.

SUICIDE
There is a very high suicide rate among elderly white men which appears to be directly related to depressive reactions and ill health. Suicide attempts are more successful among the older adult than the

young, and the methods used show the seriousness of intent (hanging, shooting, and drowning).

NUTRITION

Malnutrition in the elderly is a frequent cause of acute brain syndrome, which is reversible with proper diet. Nutritional problems in the elderly arise for many reasons, including apathy, depression, loneliness, lack of money, inability to get out and shop and lack of understanding of good nutrition. Nursing intervention in nutritional problems can bring very gratifying results with little effort, some imagination and a bit of patience.

THE "OFFICIAL" VIEW

As mentioned in the introduction to this chapter, the tendency of society is to ascribe obsolescence to people as well as to things. When a citizen can no longer produce (a man work or a woman raise a family) he or she is no longer "significant" in our society. We are told that youth, vigor, beauty and high activity are necessary for "real life." We are told by various groups that age 60 to 65 is old, 40 to 60 is middle age (on the decline), no one over 30 is to be trusted, and those under 18 aren't "dry behind the ears" yet. This narrows our active adult life down to age 18 to 30. This is how old the "beautiful people" are. This is how old everybody should be (or look). This is when we are most sexy. Heaven help those who zip through the 18 to 30 years without realizing that they are in the prime of life!

This "official American view" has been invented by a very few, distributed to everyone, and may have brought more misery and despair to more people than any other single fiction in history. Programs for the elderly are often cast in depressing humanitarian or utilitarian terms with an eye on the "official view." With medicine increasing the life span and automation reducing the age of retirement, there are increasing numbers of "them" (the elderly) who must be "dealt with." Within the parameters of the prevailing view the helping professions are beginning to think about the elderly. This is not enough. An alternate view is essential if we are to plan our own lives in a more hopeful and meaningful way and if we are really to help the older adult.

THE CHANGING POPULATION OF THE ELDERLY

As indicated in Table 12-1, the concept of just what "elderly" means is not based on physiobiologic principles but on socioeconomic factors. We all know people in their 70's and 80's who we say are "young" in their outlook, interests and involvement. They are witty, delightful, thoughtful and wise. Their views on people and the times are more than just interesting, they are valuable. On the other hand, we have seen patients who are "old" at 40. Defining "elderly" is difficult.

The Retirement Revolution

Officially, however, the elderly are all those aged 65 and up. This arbitrary figure was determined as the retirement age for Social Security purposes in 1933. The trend in retirement age is now moving steadily downward. Today some union contracts set retirement at age 55. More and more people seek retirement when they are still young enough to enjoy their leisure. Will the official definition of elderly be adjusted downwards to include age 55 or will a new definition taking function into account appear? Whichever the case, more people are joining the ranks of the retired at younger ages and inheriting many of the social and economic problems that formerly troubled only those much older.

On the other end of the scale, the "older elderly" (80 and above) are also increasing in numbers, due primarily to better health care. The result of both trends is a gradual increase in the total number of retired older persons in society.

Educational Level

Of the 20 million over age 65 in America today, 50 percent have had little education beyond elementary school. In 25 years from now the elderly population will almost all have had at least a high school education. Will this change the characteristics of the group? Will the broader educational base give the new elderly more options, more versatility in dealing with their problems?

Political Groups

Conservative groups such as the "Golden Age Clubs" and radical ones like the "Gray Panthers" are rapidly proliferating. They are both increasing the group consciousness of the older adult. Combined with the present trend towards more Federal support to the elderly, what effect will increased politicization of older persons have on their financial well being? Will the near-poverty of so many of our aged today, the cause of so much of their distress, gradually diminish?

CASE STUDY

We have repeatedly emphasized the importance for the nurse who plans to work with the elderly to rid herself of society's distorted picture and to lean heavily in a direction opposite from that of the prevailing view so that the elderly will get an even break. The following is an example of the multiple problems that the aged present, as well as the tendency to misdiagnose because of prejudice.

John P, age 63, came to the emergency room of the general hospital on his own. He quickly (without meaning to) convinced the intern, the nurse and the ward clerk that he was "crazy" and they called the mental health center for a psychiatric consultation (read "consultation" to mean "take him away").

Miss Smith responded to the call and found Mr. P sitting in a chair in a tiny room off the accident ward. The early part of the conversation went like this:

Miss S: "Hello Mr. P, I'm Miss Smith."

Mr. P "Oh, I feel okay."

Miss S: "I understand you came in alone. What has been troubling you?"

Mr. P: "Yes, I can get home, if I have the carfare."

Mr. P was wearing a hearing aid, Miss S checked it, found it wasn't operating and sent out for new batteries.

The sort of "para-logical" conversation quoted here is often seen in partially deaf, elderly persons who do not want to admit to their deafness and in an attempt to be cooperative will answer the question they think you asked without ever really hearing it.

While waiting for the batteries, Miss Smith tried other ways of communicating with Mr. P. He was illiterate, unable either to read or to write. A little sign language showed that he was hungry and a tray was sent for.

Mr. P had moderately severe ptosis of the left eyelid and paralysis of lateral gaze in his right eye resulting in severe and constant internal strabismus on the right. This combination made vision very difficult, as well as giving Mr. P the appearance of being peculiar or strange. Mr. P's dentures were ill-fitting and clacked together when he tried to speak, at times almost falling out of his mouth. His speech was barely understandable.

By midafternoon the hearing aid was operating and the following history was secured. Mr. P had come to the hospital because he had begun to experience impotence and was afraid he would lose his girlfriend (age 62). He had thought that this was because he wasn't physically active enough, so he tried to get a job as a church janitor. He was unable to obtain work because of his inability to communicate, his strange appearance and his avoidance of situations in which rejection and hurt to his pride were likely. His life became increasingly isolated as he could no longer be understood, or understand. He could not read or write, his vision was impaired, he could not hear, and his speech was distorted by ill-fitting dentures. His retreat into isolation, his lowered self-esteem, and his impotence were all the result of his impossible situation. He was a reject. He had become obsolescent. He was a "thing."

The geriatric team consisting of the nurse, the psychiatrist and the student nurse took Mr. P home to look over the situation, and found his girlfriend (whom they called Mrs. P) also in need of some help, primarily nutritional.

A month later, Mr. and Mrs. P came to a social gathering given by the geriatric service, and they both looked and felt well. The services that had been provided were:

(1) Dental care for both Mr. and Mrs. P.

(2) Hearing aid repairs for Mr. P.

(3) Ophthalmologic consultation for Mr. P.

(4) Home health aid service two days a week to help with shopping and food planning.

(5) Contact on an ongoing basis with the P family by means of home visits and invitations to have them come to the socials that were held at the center on a regular basis.

The end result? Most important to Mr. P—increased self-esteem, better appearance, improved communication, less isolation, loneliness and despair, and a resolution of the impotence. Most important to society—two elderly people, not senile or insane in any sense, were enabled to continue their independent existence in the community.

THE NEEDS OF THE ELDERLY

Elderly people need love and attention, a comfortable place to live, congenial social activities, ease of inexpensive transportation (to stores, centers for the aged, doctors and hospitals), a nutritious diet, abundant and freely given medical treatment and medical maintenance, friends, engaging activities and relationships with persons genuinely interested in knowing and listening to them, hope for the immediate future and the freedom to reflect on the process of dying, and acceptance and support of their desire for partial disengagement from high-level interaction. Few need mental health care *per se*. Almost all need a champion, a spokesman, an advocate—in short, an ombudsman.

The older adult needs what everyone else in society needs plus some special consideration of his special circumstances.

Under the best of all possible circumstances the elderly live in their own place with easy access by telephone and transportation to their neighbors, friends and family; they have an interested family doctor who visits them regularly (once every week or two) and advises them on matters of health, nutrition and medication; they have financial security through some combination of income, social security, or insurance; they enjoy themselves and are well aware that they have traded some pep for wisdom, and wouldn't have it any other way.

When one or another of these needs is no longer able to be met in the "best possible" way, social agencies and services must fill the gap to keep the older person healthy and functioning in the community.

For many, the visiting nurse service has done a magnificent job in serving the elderly, and like other forms of public health nursing it has taken a broad view of its role in the delivery of care.

In many communities "meals on wheels" service is available to give the elderly and disabled at least one hot cooked meal a day, served in their own home.

Many transportation companies give cut-rate fares to Medicare recipients.

Mental health centers are latecomers to the scene of helping the elderly. If they take the position that their job is the delivery of mental health services, and they do not define their role too narrowly, they can find great satisfaction in working out the problems of the elderly and enjoy cordial relationships with other community workers.

It is difficult to predict the kind of situation the nurse will encounter in a particular mental health center regarding services for the older adult. A few have very sophisticated geriatric departments. Most have virtually no services for the elderly at all. The trend is toward increasing Federal expenditures to stimulate the establishment of comprehensive programs for the elderly, with mental health centers coordinating the programs.

It is exciting and rewarding work. Experience with the older adult is of great value in all fields of adult mental health.

REFERENCES

1. *Physical and Mental Health.* 1971 White House Conference on Aging. Washington, D.C.: U. S. Government Printing Office, 1971. p. 53.
2. *Ibid.,* p. 49.
3. Working with Older People, a Guide to Practice, Volume 2. Washington, D.C.: U. S. Department of Health, Education, and Welfare, 1970. p. 6
4. Physical and Mental Health, p. 49.
5. Working with Older People, p. 7.
6. Physical and Mental Health, p. 49.
7. Working with Older People, p. 7.
8. *Ibid.,* p. 44.
9. *Ibid.,* p. 15.
10. *Ibid.,* p. 34.
11. Physical and Mental Health, p. 49.

FURTHER READING

Masters, William H. and Virginia E. Johnson, Human Sexual Response. Boston: Little, Brown, 1966.
Toffler, Alvin. Future Shock. New York: Random House, 1970.
The Aged and Community Mental Health: A Guide to Program Development. Vol. 8, Report 81. New York: Committee on Aging, 1971.

13

Social Aspects of Mental Health

CASE STUDY

A 45-year-old mother of nine children came to the community mental health center following hospitalization for a suspected suicide attempt. She had been found unconscious by her 14-year-old daughter on the kitchen floor with the oven door open and the gas jets on.

The patient presented as a proud, concerned, but overwhelmed woman who readily admitted to feeling depressed over her impossible living situation. She denied a suicide attempt, explaining that she had attempted to use the kitchen stove to heat the downstairs of her home because her welfare check had been "delayed by computer breakdown" (this was verified by her caseworker) and she was unable to purchase coal to heat her home. Apparently the flame had been extinguished from the jets and gas fumes permeated the confined kitchen area, causing her to pass out. She was resentful that the attending physician had suspected she would "do myself in and leave my kids to the welfare people." In the course of emergency interview (because of the suspected suicide attempt) it was learned that Mrs. L (the patient) had been in therapy at the community mental health center off and on for three years because of depression. Therapy had been terminated several months prior to the latest referral because, according to her therapist's notes, "Mrs. L has adjusted to the reality of her living situation." The patient had by no means accepted the "reality" of her situation, and was actively trying to cut through the incredible red tape of the many city welfare and social agencies with whom she had contact in order to secure better housing for herself and her children. (The euphemistic termination note of the therapist could indicate the therapist's reluctance or inability to assist the patient in solving her social problems, and the patient's resistance to accept psychotherapy in lieu of safer, sounder housing for her family.)

The patient had been seen by several clinic therapists over a three-year period. She had several "diagnostic" labels applied to her "symptoms:" anxiety neurosis, neurotic depression, schizo-affective depressed, and schizoid personality.* The state had reimbursed the clinic for her "therapy" sessions (one hour once a week) at the rate of $15.00 per session. She had been seen almost 100 times in the three-year period, and had had one brief (eight days) psychiatric hospitalization because of her "depression." The state had thus spent over 2,000 dollars for Mrs. L's therapy, and yet her symptoms remained unchanged. She was depressed, frustrated, anxious and angry. And she refused to accept the finality of her situation.

Mrs. L had six minor children living at home with her. Of the older four, two were married and lived separately, and two had been placed in Quaker boarding schools where they qualified because they were "disadvantaged but deserving". The children had several different fathers, and Mrs. L explained she had never married because she felt none of them had been responsible, as she felt she was. She had worked intermittently as a domestic, but had for the most part been on welfare during her adult life. She had high aspirations for her children, and she was determined to prevent their inheritance of her life style. Her depression, in a sense, resulted from the double-bind of her situation: She was chastised by her welfare worker for having too many children (she had been encouraged earlier to have an abortion and tubal ligation), punished by the state by frequent delays in her welfare check, informed by the schools her children attended that academic success was not expected of them because of their "circumstances" (as an explanation for the school's suggestion that the children take a vocational curriculum, not academic), and subject to improbable and impossible external interference in almost every aspect of her and her family's life. But as she attempted to change her environment by securing better housing and improving her children's education by relocating near better schools, thereby reducing the anxiety and fear she and her children suffered because of their woefully inadequate, rat- and vermin-infested housing, she encountered the brickbats of the system. The message communicated to Mrs. L was: stay put, stay down, don't rock the boat and don't complain. In a uniquely intuitive way this patient suggested that she felt "the system" (her apt descrip-

*An indication of both the subjective interpretation of symptoms and the inadequacy of the mental disorder diagnostic system.

tion of all the agencies she had to deal with in her daily survival) had been willing to pay the community mental health center to provide psychotherapy for her as a means of helping her accept and like her life. It was difficult to disagree with her point.

The first interview was to assess her situation, sort out the problems she presented and make some decision about what the next step would be. Mrs. L insisted she had made no suicide attempt. At this point, the therapist's decision that Mrs. L was correct was intuitive, and reflected trust in the patient's own assessment of her situation. She wanted help if that was available; she had not given up even though she felt depressed. It would have been inappropriate if she had felt other than depressed!

The next session was scheduled for a few days later and Mrs. L seemed genuinely pleased when it was suggested that the children be present, and that the therapist would come to her home.

Checking out the center records on Mrs. L and contacting her welfare caseworker supported the impression that most of the psychiatric symptoms she presented were in reaction to her social problems. In some strange way the caseworker suggested that no "push" was being made to resolve Mrs. L's housing situation because she was "mentally ill" and "would probably not be a good risk" for relocation in a housing project.

When visited in her home Mrs. L was more relaxed, indicating she felt hopeful that "finally somebody's going to listen to my side of the story." It was readily apparent that the relationship between Mrs. L and her children was warm, natural, and indicative of openness and trust. The overwhelming concern of all the L's was their housing situation. Mrs. L had indicated alarm that her eight- and nine-year-old sons had begun to "wet their beds"; the boys explained they were afraid to get up to go to the toilet at night because "the rats might get us." By the end of the second interview two facts were established:

1. Mrs. L had a close, reciprocal and healthy relationship with her children, thus obviating the need for family therapy intervention;

2. Social pathology rather than psychopathology was the major problem of this family.

The next move could have been referral of this resolute lady back to her social service agency contacts, but that would have perpetuated the circular nature of her problem and compounded her double-bind situation.

At this juncture, Mrs. L was asked to make some com-

ments on her situation, its prospects for change and the pre-
requisites she felt necessary to bring about a change. Very
quickly she indicated that she had found a redevelopment
house on her own, that it would "fit us perfect," having two
bathrooms, five bedrooms and a small fenced yard. She had
the names of necessary people to call readily available, the
date the house could be moved into, familiarity with the
neighborhood schools and the total monthly cost for rent
and utilities. She *did not* have the 200 dollars for security
payment and moving expenses, and she doubted she ever
would. Despite careful budgeting, the L family existed from
check to check, and there was no hope of saving the needed
money. Because she received welfare she was ineligible to
make loans, have charge accounts, checking accounts or other
of the minor conveniences everyone else takes for granted.°

Impressed with the tenacity and motivation of Mrs. L,
and again trusting the "feel" of the patient and situation, the
innovative idea decided on was to assist the patient in securing a bank loan to cover moving expenses. Contact with a
local bank which advertised itself as concerned with financial
problems of the poor was helpful in that a loan could be
made to Mrs. L if the therapist agreed to cosign. The risk
seemed minimal when compared to the alternative. Because
the risk was personal, no permission was necessary from the
community mental health center. But, if the plan was successful, then perhaps the center would be interested in establishing
a contingency fund for similar use by other patients.

The loan was secured, the patient and her family were
able to relocate, and after 18 months the patient had not
manifested any clinical symptoms of depression. She had been
faithful in repaying the loan, although she was informed by
the bank that she would not be able to borrow again without
a cosigner. (Even her remarkable repayment record was not
credited to her, and she could not establish a credit rating
because the loan had been cosigned. Mrs. L's comment about
the inequity of this was that "the system sure has a lot of
power!" Double-binding is an operational tactic of individuals, families and society.

Mrs. L was able to call the therapist on a p.r.n. basis,
which she did, and when she seemed upset or concerned
about a problem she was encouraged to come in and talk.
Any attempt to encourage dependency of this patient on the
therapist or community mental health center was avoided,
although her initial desire to continue the relationship with

---

°In order to pay bills it was necessary for Mrs. L to spend 35 cents for a money
order (bank checks are 10 cents) or to go in person to each business to whom she
owed money, using both time and money for carfare.

someone who "can solve my problems" had to be worked out after the housing problem had been negotiated.

The main point we wish to demonstrate by this case study is the fallacy of evaluating a patient's (or his family's) function, symptoms or dynamics without considering the social factors involved in each instance, especially when the identified patient is a parent and the family income is at the poverty level. Minuchin et al.[1] cited a study of mental illness prevalence in a random sampling study of a large northern city which we find very true in community mental health center practice:

> . . . it appears that on the whole lowered economic status is associated with more psychoses. How much of this is cause and how much effect we cannot state from our data. It is quite likely that both mechanisms are operative here. A certain number (of individuals) have probably been forced into the lower economic status because of psychosis, and it is also probable that because of a number of factors associated with low income a sizable group of . . . individuals have been forced into this psychotic group.

The nurse practitioner in a community mental health center would recognize the patient and the situation described in the example above. They are both all too familiar, particularly in inner city catchment areas designated by government agencies to "handle" mental health problems in a given community. The nurse new to a community mental health facility must quickly learn to distinguish between social pathology and psychopathology. She will be called upon to evaluate, diagnose, intervene and treat in both situations, and she will find to her dismay and frustration that frequently there is no discrete demarcation between them.

Community psychiatry should be practiced on three levels of prevention:

1. Primary prevention, by elimination of the causes of specific psychiatric disorders and by intervention to prevent the spread of certain disorders;
2. Secondary prevention, by early case finding, psychiatric evaluation and active treatment; and
3. Rehabilitation that focuses on the minimizing of the disabling effects of chronic or severe mental illness by well planned and accessible after-care treatment.

For the most part, community mental health has succeeded in at least part of its original mandate: secondary prevention. Treatment is available and in most community mental health centers it is readily and easily obtainable. In areas where the population density is great (urban) or where the geographic area is large (rural) there are frequently extensions of the home center which reach into the community and are commonly called "satellite" clinics, "walk-in" clinics or "coping" clinics.

Their chief purpose is to increase the secondary prevention aspect of community mental health and in that respect they are successful. Additionally, such center extensions are able to offer a more personalized service which is useful to patients who have often experienced impersonal attention in larger and more distant mental health institutions. However, the community mental health focus today remains an essentially treatment-oriented movement. The case study which opened this chapter clearly demonstrates that "the system," of which community psychiatry is a part, is not responsive enough to the social factors which so often result in mental illness. The idea of community-based mental health facilities with an emphasis on primary prevention is perhaps still futuristic. Certainly, as we know from experience, it is very costly.

In community mental health practice it is frequent that the individual seeking treatment, or identified as needing treatment, represents "the symptom" of social injustice, unresponsiveness and neglect. That is not surprising. Many centers, as mentioned earlier, are located in urban ghetto areas and it is known that family disorganization and psychopathology occur with greater frequency in these areas. Overcrowding, both within the home and community, and economic insecurity (poverty) are two common problems of which patients coming to urban community mental health centers complain. These social pressures, and the frustration of being caught in an unresponsive system, predispose some to impulsive acting-out. When living is reduced to enduring, the exercise of self-control does not seem desirable or even possible. Gratification of whatever type is to be experienced *now* and not postponed. Naturally, these attitudes clash with established social values and with the law. When this occurs the end result may be referral to a mental health clinic for evaluation and treatment. The rationale seems to be that social problems *are* mental health problems and that psychiatric treatment is a solution. Neither is true.

The community mental health nurse should have knowledge and experience in clinical psychiatry. Beyond that she should make every effort to acquire some knowledge of the laws regulating mental illness and social institutions, governmental process (which is frequently a euphemism for red tape) and community organization process. It is in her understanding of such processes, in conjunction with her skill in "using" them, that she will be able to intervene more effectively in many of the situations patients seeking her help will identify, or she for them, as the "real" problem.

In more traditional psychiatric practice the nurse, and her non-nurse colleagues, function in rather specifically defined roles: psychologists are involved in research and testing, social workers assist with money or social problems, psychiatrists prescribe medication and treatment (and generally have more say about who does what, and for what reasons) and administrators administer. The nurse, in such settings, cares for the patient more directly and concretely than any other professional, although her care may be limited because of her role definition.

In the less traditional but not yet ideal community mental health setting the nurse will have more direct influence, if she can and will accept it, based on the quality of the intervention she makes on behalf of the individuals she will treat. Treatment is not traditional in such a setting. Neither are the complex and varied problems one sees.

SPECIFIC PROBLEM AREAS:

Poverty

It is probably true that money doesn't guarantee happiness or success; at least we are told that is so. However, it is also probably true that more people are unhappy, unsuccessful and unhealthy because they lack money than for any other general reason.

It is not possible, as the case of Mrs. L points out, to endure the constant struggle of "being without" and "doing without" and not experience anger, frustration and despair. There are stoics and spartan types who choose to conduct their lives at a subsistence level. That is admirable; that is their *choice*. We can wonder about the motives of people who make such a choice. We can be curious about their life style, envy or emulate them (though few of us do), laugh at them, label them (and we do), and speculate about their achievements, but we do not need to help them change. Choice implies freedom. When people *choose* to live without the comforts and necessities most of us expect, seek and take for granted, then presumably, they have what they want and if not they can make another choice. That is the way things should be. People, all people, should have the option to choose the life style they feel is right and proper for them. Poverty denies choice, limits freedom and restricts options.

Most people choose not to be poor and to do without. The "American Way" is to produce, to possess and to consume. Somehow, poor people violate society's concept of the right way, and in so doing are punished, just as Mrs. L felt she was punished. She was correct in her feelings and intuition about what had happened to her, and her expectations about what would continue to happen to her and her children unless she persisted in her fight against the labels and "pigeon holes" she was pressured into.

Community mental health and public health nurses, probably more than nurses in other areas of practice, are familiar with the effects of poverty on mental and physical health *in situ*.

Poverty is oppressive to the body, the mind and the spirit. It causes neglect of physical care because there is never enough money to have or to *prevent* physical disease. Everything must wait "until I have the money." The wait, which is usually interminable, creates mental pressures: fear, anxiety, increased tension and eventually apathy. Poverty necessitates indifference and although indifference is not recognized as a legitimate *defense mechanism,* it is. The nurse who routinely interprets such indifference as "I don't care" is insensitive to the probable meaning, which is "I can't care." Poor people don't have an *esprit de corps*. They often despair that things will improve or that things will change. They learn, in the pervasiveness and constancy of their poverty, that they must always "settle for." The ambiguities and obfuscations of the myriad agencies they are evaluated by and assigned to frequently confuse them. The community mental health nurse is in a unique position to intervene in their behalf to seek clarification of agency policy and exceptions to "the rule" when that is needed. Poor people who retreat into mental illness to escape from their social milieu and endless hassles, frequently need an advocate as much as they need medication, hospitalization, or psychotherapy. The nurse who defines her role as a psychotherapist must realize that in the community mental health center setting that is a less discrete and less definable term. The nurse therapist, nurse practitioner, nurse clinician, or whatever she chooses to label herself (or is labelled) cannot be therapeutic if she neglects or does not attempt to treat the social problems she will so often encounter in mentally disabled patients who are poor. The opportunities for creativity, innovation, and success may be limited in a general way by the policies and financial constraints of a community mental health center, but such opportunities are always inherent in the individual transactions the nurse will have with *her* patients.

Housing

"... We proceed to a guarantee that must come from society: spatial arrangements must be such that minimum distortion, psychological or physiological, may inhibit or divert the development of society's members. But what are these arrangements? And how much does overcrowding as such distort us?"

There is little doubt, after much study, that overcrowding of any sort is unhealthy and impairs human growth, development and potential. Crowded classrooms do not enhance learning. Crowded highways are more dangerous even for careful drivers. Crowding of any sort is often prohibited in public places by legal restrictions: number of beds in a hospital, people in an elevator, theater, auditorium, vehicle, etc. Crowding is not safe, is not desirable, is to be avoided.

It is not uncommon, in rural but more often in urban areas, that an individual seeking treatment for a mental health problem in a community center will identify his living arrangement as inadequate. Frequently, the inadequacy of the housing is in its disrepair, neglect and deterioration, as well as in its spatial inadequacy for the families or individuals who inhabit it.

Many older people, poor people and mentally or physically disabled people spend their lives in single-room apartments, transient hotels and rooming houses, or boarding homes. Privacy is an impossible luxury for such individuals, and in their attempts to survive in such situations they often become anxious and depressed.

The nurse practitioner in a community mental health center setting should become familiar with the varieties and conditions of housing in the community served by her mental health center. Knowing what a certain address means in terms of neighborhood circumstances can be helpful in making a diagnosis about the problems and situation presented by a patient.

Because hospitalization is often sought as a relief from overcrowded and impossible permanent living arrangements it is both useful and necessary for the nurse to develop contacts, on her own, with area residents who are able and willing to provide temporary housing for people whose chief problem may be their need to "get away" from a too cramped or volatile situation.

When temporary solutions are not possible or feasible, for whatever reason, it is incumbent on the community mental health nurse to become actively involved in assisting a patient, or his family, to relocate; that is also psychotherapy, if not by precise definition. The nurse in the L case example used skills not generally taught in a nursing education curriculum. She was a successful change agent for the L family by her willingness to extend herself beyond her accepted nurse's role and in doing so she enhanced her professional competence.

REFERENCES

1. Ardrey, R. The Social Contract ... New York: Athenium, 1970. p. 220.

FURTHER READING

Panzetta, A. F. Community Mental Health. Philadelphia: Lea and Febiger, 1971.
Bellak, L. Handbook of Community Psychiatry and Community Mental Health. New York: Grune and Stratton, 1964.

Mental Status Examination

This form is used for the final organization of the material of observation and evaluation of the patient. It is not to be followed for the rigid structuring of an interview, nor should it merely contain the immediate illegible scratch notes.

No.   Name   Date   Examiner

1. Attitude, appearance and general behavior:

2. Affect, mood and emotional responsiveness:

3. Stream of mental activity: (to include a sufficiently long sample of continuous flow of talk to demonstrate the characteristics of talk and of the patient's thinking.)

4. Mental trend: (this section includes specific description of the content of the patient's spontaneous and responsive verbalizations to demonstrate special preoccupations and experiences and underlying dynamic factors. Emotional reactions which occur during these discussions should be included as well as the character of convictions, projections and special concerns.)

5. Orientation:
   Time:
   Place:
   Persons present:
   Self:

6. Memory:

    (a) Remote past:
    (b) Recent past:
    (c) Immediate impressions:
    (d) General grasp and recall:

    A cowboy/ from Arizona/ went to San Francisco/ with his dog/ which he left/ at a friend's/ while he purchased/ a new suit of clothes./ Dressed finely,/ he went back/ to the dog,/ whistled to him,/ called him by name,/ and patted him./ But the dog would have nothing to do with him,/ in his new hat/ and coat,/ but gave a mournful/ howl./ Coaxing was of no effect,/ so the cowboy went away/ and donned his old garments,/ whereupon the dog, immediately/ showed his wild joy/ on seeing his master/ as he thought he ought to be./

(Patient's recall of story verbatim.)

Calif. for his dog .... while went shopping .... clothes .... dog accepted him as ? should be

Total Score...................

P.H.

No.	Name	Date	Examiner

7. Attention and Concentration:
    (a) Digit Span

Digits Forward	Digits Backward
Score:	Score:
3 8 6	2 5
6 1 2	6 3
3 4 1 7	5 7 4
6 1 5 8	2 5 9
8 4 2 3 9	7 2 9 6
5 2 1 8 6	8 4 1 3
3 8 9 1 7 4	4 1 6 2 7 ✓
7 9 6 4 8 3	9 7 8 5 2
5 1 7 4 2 3 8	1 6 5 2 9 8
9 8 5 2 1 6 3	3 6 7 1 9 4
1 6 4 5 9 7 6 3	8 5 9 2 3 4 2
2 9 7 6 3 1 5 4	4 5 7 9 2 8 1
5 3 8 7 1 2 4 6 9 ✓	6 9 1 6 3 2 5 8
4 2 6 9 1 7 8 3 5	3 1 7 9 5 4 8 2

(b) Serial subtraction

I want to see how well you can subtract by 3's. Begin at 40 and subtract 3 until you reach 1; like this, $40 - 37 - 34 - - - - -$

8. General Intellectual Evaluation:

31
28
25
22
19
16

(a) General Information

How many days are there in a week?

How many things make a dozen?

What do we celebrate on the fourth of July?

What animal does wool come from?

Where does the sun set?

What is a barometer?

Who invented the airplane? *Wright Bros.*

What do we get turpentine from? *✓*

What is a hieroglyphic?

What is a prime number?

Who discovered the South Pole?

8. (b) Calculations

Compute 1½ years' interest on $200 at 4%.

If 5 times X equals 20, how much is X? *4*

(c) Symbolization

Differences between abstract words (idleness and laziness; poverty and misery; character and reputation; irresponsible and incapable.)

Explain the proverb: *never settles down - always*

A rolling stone gathers no moss. *on move.*

Too many cooks spoil the broth. *too many people spoil*

No use crying over spilt milk. *Something*

(d) Reasoning and judgment

Why should a promise be kept? *more than one human*

Why are laws necessary? — *nec. to hold soc. struct.*

Why is it better to build a house of brick than of wood?

9. Insight: *brick more durable*

10. Summary:

APPENDIX ▌▌

Diagnostic Nomenclature of the American Psychiatric Association

I MENTAL RETARDATION

310.	Borderline
311.	Mild
312.	Moderate
313.	Severe
314.	Profound
315.	Unspecified

With each: Following or associated with

.0	Infection or intoxication
.1	Trauma or physical agent
.2	Disorders of metabolism, growth or nutrition
.3	Gross brain disease (postnatal)
.4	Unknown prenatal influence
.5	Chromosomal abnormality
.6	Prematurity
.7	Major psychiatric disorder
.8	Psychosocial (environmental) deprivation
.9	Other condition

II ORGANIC BRAIN SYNDROMES (OBS)

A PSYCHOSES

Senile and presenile dementia

290.0	Senile dementia
290.1	Presenile dementia

Alcoholic psychosis

291.0	Delirium tremens
291.1	Korsakov's psychosis
291.2	Other alcoholic hallucinosis
291.3	Alcohol paranoid state
291.4	Acute alcohol intoxication
291.5	Alcoholic deterioration
291.6	Pathological intoxication
291.9	Other alcoholic psychosis

Psychosis associated with intracranial infection

292.0	General paralysis
292.1	Syphilis of central nervous system
292.2	Epidemic encephalitis
292.3	Other and unspecified encephalitis
292.9	Other intracranial infection

Psychosis associated with other cerebral condition

293.0	Cerebral arteriosclerosis
293.1	Other cerebrovascular disturbance
293.2	Epilepsy
293.3	Intracranial neoplasm
293.4	Degenerative disease of the CNS
293.5	Brain trauma
293.9	Other cerebral condition

Psychosis associated with other physical condition

294.0	Endocrine disorder
294.1	Metabolic and nutritional disorder
294.2	Systemic infection
294.3	Drug or poison intoxication (other than alcohol)

294.4 Childbirth
294.8 Other and unspecified physical condition

B NONPSYCHOTIC OBS
309.0 Intracranial infection
309.13 Alcohol (simple drunkenness)
309.14 Other drug, poison or systemic intoxication
309.2 Brain trauma
309.3 Circulatory disturbance
309.4 Epilepsy
309.5 Disturbance of metabolism, growth, or nutrition
309.6 Senile or presenile brain disease
309.7 Intracranial neoplasm
309.8 Degenerative disease of the CNS
309.9 Other physical condition

III PSYCHOSES NOT ATTRIBUTED TO PHYSICAL CONDITIONS LISTED PREVIOUSLY
Schizophrenia
295.0 Simple
295.1 Hebephrenic
295.2 Catatonic
295.23 Catatonic type, excited
295.24 Catatonic type, withdrawn
295.3 Paranoid
295.4 Acute schizophrenic episode
295.5 Latent
295.6 Residual
295.7 Schizo-affective
295.73 Schizo-affective, excited
295.74 Schizo-affective, depressed
295.8 Childhood
295.90 Chronic undifferentiated
295.99 Other schizophrenia

Major affective disorders
296.0 Involutional melancholia
296.1 Manic-depressive illness, manic
296.2 Manic-depressive illness, depressed
296.3 Manic-depressive illness, circular
296.33 Manic-depressive, circular, manic
296.34 Manic-depressive, circular, depressed

296.8 Other major affective disorder
Paranoid states
297.0 Paranoia
297.1 Involutional paraphrenia
297.9 Other paranoid state
Other psychoses
298.0 Psychotic depressive reaction

IV NEUROSES
300.0 Anxiety
300.1 Hysterical
300.13 Hysterical, conversion type
300.14 Hysterical, dissociative type
300.2 Phobic
300.3 Obsessive compulsive
300.4 Depressive
300.5 Neurasthenic
300.6 Depersonalization
300.7 Hypochondriacal
300.8 Other neurosis

V PERSONALITY DISORDERS AND CERTAIN OTHER NON-PSYCHOTIC MENTAL DISORDERS
Personality disorders
301.0 Paranoid
301.1 Cyclothymic
301.2 Schizoid
301.3 Explosive
301.4 Obsessive compulsive
301.5 Hysterical
301.6 Asthenic
301.7 Antisocial
301.81 Passive-aggressive
301.82 Inadequate
301.89 Other specified types
Sexual deviation
302.0 Homosexuality
302.1 Fetishism
302.2 Pedophilia
302.3 Transvestitism
302.4 Exhibitionism
302.5 Voyeurism
302.6 Sadism
302.7 Masochism
302.8 Other sexual deviation
Alcoholism
303.0 Episodic excessive drinking
303.1 Habitual excessive drinking
303.2 Alcohol addiction
303.9 Other alcoholism

Drug dependence

304.0 Opium, opium alkaloids and their derivatives

304.1 Synthetic analgesics with morphine-like effects

304.2 Barbiturates

304.3 Other hypnotics and sedatives or "tranquilizers"

304.4 Cocaine

304.5 Cannabis sativa (hashish, marihuana)

304.6 Other psychostimulants

304.7 Hallucinogens

304.8 Other drug dependence

VI PSYCHOPHYSIOLOGIC DISORDERS

305.0 Skin

305.1 Musculoskeletal

305.2 Respiratory

305.3 Cardiovascular

305.4 Hemic and lymphatic

305.5 Gastro-intestinal

305.6 Genito-urinary

305.7 Endocrine

305.8 Organ of special sense

305.9 Other type

VII SPECIAL SYMPTOMS

306.0 Speech disturbance

306.1 Specific learning disturbance

306.2 Tic

306.3 Other psychomotor disorder

306.4 Disorders of sleep

306.5 Feeding disturbance

306.6 Enuresis

306.7 Encopresis

306.8 Cephalagia

306.9 Other special symptom

VIII TRANSIENT SITUATIONAL DISTURBANCES

307.0 Adjustment reaction of infancy

307.1 Adjustment reaction of childhood

307.2 Adjustment reaction of adolescence

307.3 Adjustment reaction of adult life

307.4 Adjustment reaction of late life

IX BEHAVIOR DISORDERS OF CHILDHOOD AND ADOLESCENCE

308.0 Hyperkinetic reaction

308.1 Withdrawing reaction

308.2 Overanxious reaction

308.3 Runaway reaction

308.4 Unsocialized aggressive reaction

308.5 Group delinquent reaction

308.9 Other reaction

X CONDITIONS WITHOUT MANIFEST PSYCHIATRIC DISORDER AND NON-SPECIFIC CONDITIONS

Social maladjustment without manifest psychiatric disorder

316.0 Marital maladjustment

316.1 Social maladjustment

316.2 Occupational maladjustment

316.3 Dyssocial behavior

316.9 Other social maladjustment

Nonspecific conditions

317 Nonspecific conditions

No Mental Disorder

318 No mental disorder

XI NONDIAGNOSTIC TERMS FOR ADMINISTRATIVE USE

319.0 Diagnosis deferred

319.1 Boarder

319.2 Experiment only

319.9 Other

Community Mental
Health Act

The Community Mental Health Act of 1964, mandates that a community mental health center should, by its philosophy and design, be accessible to the community it serves, and include a minimum of five basic services:
1. Inpatient treatment.
2. Outpatient treatment.
3. Partial hospitalization (day or night programs).
4. Emergency services, on a 24-hour-a-day basis.
5. Consultation and Education services to community agencies, groups and individuals.

There is provision for five additional services which, while not prerequisite, are desirable from the standpoint of function, implementation, and continuity of the five basic services:
6. Diagnostic services.
7. Rehabilitation.
8. Pre-care and after-care.
9. Training programs for professionals and nonprofessionals.
10. Research and evaluation.

When a center has all ten services operational then it is usually known as a comprehensive community mental health center. However, adjectives can be misleading; quantity does not assure quality. To provide all the services in some incomplete or shallow fashion, as occasionally occurs, is no service to the community. The five services mandated should be fully and qualitatively functional before other services are added. The basic services are basic—and in a sense that is "where the action is," for both staff, and community residents requesting or requiring community mental health service.

According to the Community Mental Health Act a center must serve a specific area with a population of between 75,000 and 200,000. Thus, in some remote rural areas the geographic boundaries containing a minimum population may be measured in hundreds of square miles, while in densely populated urban areas a maximum population may exist in less than 100 square blocks. Once the population determines the geographic boundaries a community mental health center is to serve, a "catchment" area is designated. The term catchment area is borrowed from the phrase used to describe reservoirs which catch water runoff after storms. In urban areas underground sewers are also divided into catchment areas. Considering the history of society's treatment of its mentally ill, one is tempted to speculate on the rationale for such a choice of terms!

In a large rural area the community mental health center is not always in close proximity to area residents wanting or needing services. However, to be accessible, travel time to the center should not exceed one hour.

All community mental health centers are not the same. One popular idea is that those centers which originate with community support, and reflect the needs defined by community leaders, are more successful. While this may be so, and many communities feel only they know what is good for their community, this has not been validated. Neither has it been proven that centers which develop without close consultation with the community or popular community support will be less successful. Federal law establishing the priority for delivering services is the same for all centers. All community residents who need care, regardless of age or social-economic factors, are eligible for treatment from the community mental health center in their area.

Glossary

Addiction: Describes the compulsive use of chemical substances on which the individual has become physiologically dependent, and without which he will experience withdrawal reaction.

Affect: Refers to the mood or emotion an individual shows in response to a given situation. Affect can be described, according to its expression, as: blunted, blocked, flat, inappropriate or displaced.

Ambivalence: The coexistence of two opposing feelings toward another person, object, or idea. (Examples: love-hate, pleasure-pain, like-dislike).

Anxiety: Apprehension, tension, or uneasiness that stems from the anticipation of danger, the source of which is largely unknown or unrecognized. Primarily of intrapsychic origin, in distinction to fear, which is the emotional response to a consciously recognized and usually external threat or danger. Anxiety and fear are accompanied by similar physiologic changes. May be regarded as pathologic when present to such an extent as to interfere with effectiveness in living, achievement of desired goals or satisfactions or reasonable emotional comfort.*

Confabulation: Refers to a symptom usually seen in organic psychotic disorders (e.g., Korsokov's psychosis) in which the individual defensively attempts to "fill in" details about the past, which he cannot recall because of memory loss. Imaginary experiences are often related in a detailed and plausible fashion.

Conflict: In psychoanalytic terms, it describes the mental struggle which occurs when there are opposing impulses, drives and demands of the id, ego and super-ego.

Conjoint Therapy: Refers to the psychotherapy of couples or entire families treated together, at the same time, by the same therapist.

Covert: Implies secrecy, or hidden reasons for conscious actions or behavior.

Crisis Intervention Therapy: A type of brief psychiatric treatment in which individuals (and/or families) are assisted in their efforts to cope, and problem solve in crisis situations. The treatment approach is immediate, supportive, and direct.

Defense Mechanisms: Unconscious intrapsychic processes that are em-

---

*Entries marked with an asterisk are from American Psychiatric Association, A Psychiatric Glossary, 3rd edition. Washington, D.C.: American Psychiatric Association, 1969.

ployed to seek relief from emotional conflict and freedom from anxiety. Conscious efforts are frequently made for the same reasons, but true defense mechanisms are out of awareness (unconscious).* The common defense mechanisms are:

DEFENSE MECHANISMS

1. COMPENSATION—putting forth extra effort to achieve in the area in which there is a real or imagined deficiency.
2. CONVERSION—the unconscious expression of a mental conflict by means of a physical symptom.
3. DENIAL—treating obvious reality factors as though they do not exist because they are consciously intolerable.
4. DISPLACEMENT—transferring unacceptable feelings aroused by one object or situation to a more acceptable substitute.
5. DISSOCIATION—walling off certain areas of the personality from consciousness.
6. FANTASY—satisfying needs by day-dreaming.
7. FIXATION—never advancing the level of emotional development beyond that in which one feels comfortable.
8. IDEALIZATION—conscious or unconscious overestimation of another's attributes. e.g., hero worship.
9. IDENTIFICATION—attaching to one's self certain qualities associated with others. Operates unconsciously and is significant mechanism in super-ego development.
10. INTROJECTION—incorporating the traits of others; internalizing feelings towards others.
11. ISOLATION—separating thought and affect, allowing only the former to come to consciousness. It is a compromise mechanism.
12. PROJECTION—unconsciously attributing one's own unacceptable qualities and emotions to others.
13. RATIONALIZATION—attempting to justify or to make consciously tolerable by plausible means, feelings, behavior and motives that would otherwise be intolerable.
14. REACTION FORMATION—expressing unacceptable wishes or behavior in socially acceptable manner.
15. REGRESSION—going back to an earlier level of emotional development and organization.
16. REPRESSION—unconscious, involuntary forgetting of unacceptable or painful thoughts, impulses, feelings, or acts.
17. SUBLIMATION—directing energy from unacceptable drives into socially acceptable behavior.
18. SUBSTITUTION—unconsciously attempting to make up for a deficiency in one area by concentrating efforts in another area that is more attainable.

19. SUPPRESSION—the conscious, deliberate forgetting of unacceptable or painful thoughts, impulses, feelings, or acts.
20. SYMBOLIZATION—using an object or idea as a substitute or to represent some other object or idea.
21. UNDOING—thinking or doing one thing for the purpose of neutralizing something objectionable which was thought or done before.

Delusion: A false belief or opinion which is unreasonable and causes distortion in judgment.

Depersonalization: Feelings of unreality or strangeness concerning either the environment or the self or both.*

Double-Bind: A type of interaction, generally associated with schizophrenic families, in which one individual demands a response to a message containing mutually contradictory signals while the other is unable to respond or comment on the inconsistent and incongruous message. Best characterized by the damned if you do, damned if you don't situation.

Dyad: Refers to the relationship between two people; dyadic pair can be husband and wife, parent and child, sibling and sibling. In music it describes a chord composed of two tones.

Ego: That part of the personality, according to Freudian theory, which mediates between the primitive, pleasure-seeking instinctual drives of the id and the self-critical, prohibitive, restraining forces of the super-ego. The compromises worked out, on an unconscious level, help to resolve intrapsychic conflict by keeping thoughts, interpretations, judgments and behavior practical and efficient. The ego is directed by the reality principle, meaning it is in contact with the real world, as well as the id and super-ego. The ego develops as the individual grows. (See super-ego, id.)

Extrapyramidal Reaction: Refers to the usually reversible side effect of some of the major psychotropic drugs on the extrapyramidal system of the C.N.S. Characterized by a variety of physical signs and symptoms (similar to those seen in patients with Parkinson's disease) which include: muscular rigidity, tremors, drooling, restlessness, shuffling gait, blurred vision and other neurologic disturbances.

Family Therapy: Treatment of more than one member of the family simultaneously in the same session. The treatment may be supportive, directive, or interpretive. The assumption is that a mental disorder in one member of a family may be a manifestation of disorder in other members and in their interrelationships and functioning as a total group.*

Gestalt Psychology: The study of mental process and behavior with emphasis on a total perceptual configuration and the interrelation of component parts. Generally, refers to the "whole person" approach to assessment and treatment of psychiatric patients.

Group Therapy: Application of psychotherapeutic techniques to a group of individuals who have similar problems and are in reasonably good contact with reality, by one or more therapist. The optimal size of a group is six to ten members. As a therapy procedure it is popular because it is a versatile, economical and generally successful modality.

Hallucination: An imagined sensory perception which occurs without an external stimulus. Can be auditory, visual, or tactile. Usually occurs in psychotic disorders, but can occur in both chronic and acute organic brain disorders.

Heterosexuality: The direction of sexual interest and behavior towards persons of the opposite sex.

Homeostasis: A term borrowed from physiology meant to indicate the selfregulating intrapsychic processes which are optimal for comfort and survival.

Homosexuality: Refers to the sexual preference, attraction and relationship between two people of the same sex.

Id: In Freudian theory, the id is identified as the reservoir of psychic energy. It is guided by the pleasure principle, curbed by the ego, and is unconscious. The id wants what it wants when it wants it! (See ego, super-ego.) Babies are born with an id.

Identified Patient: Refers to the designation by the family unit of one member who is "sick," and who is identified as the patient in need of treatment. In family therapy theory the sick member of the family system who exhibits symptoms of psychopathology is regarded as a symptom of family pathology.

Illusion: A misinterpretation of the sensory stimuli, usually auditory or visual, of a real experience.

Insight: The ability of an individual to understand himself and the basis for his attitudes and behavior.

Intrapsychic: Refers to all that which takes place with in the mind (psyche).

Latent: Adjective used to describe feelings, drives, and emotions which influence behavior but remain repressed, outside of conscious thought.

Life Style: Refers to the choice each individual ultimately makes about how, where, and for what purpose he chooses to conduct his life.

L.S.D. (Lysergic acid diethylamide): A potent drug which, taken in very small quantities, produces toxic symptoms and behavior similar to certain psychoses.

Mental Status Exam: Usually refers to a formal examination of the patient's cognitive and intrapsychic functioning. Questions presented to the patient are designed to evaluate his orientation to time, place and person, intelligence, concentration, memory judgment, insight, abstract reasoning and affect. It cannot be relied upon to accurately assess the patient, and is used chiefly as a guide to conduct a psychiatric interview, or assist with a differential diagnostic problem.

Milieu: The immediate environment, both physical and social.

Motivation: Describes the individual's will and determination to persevere and succeed.

Neologism: A new word which is invented or made up by condensing other words into a new one. Typical in schizophrenia.

Neurosis: An impairment of personality development and growth which is characterized by excessive use of energy for unproductive purposes. The chief symptom in neurotic disorders is anxiety which is either felt directly or controlled by various psychologic mechanisms to produce other, subjectively distressing symptoms. Although in some of its forms and degrees it is incapacitating it does not interfere with the individual's contact with reality; psychosis implies flight from reality, neurosis an attempt to come to terms with it.

Nosology: The scientific classification of diseases.

Overt: Open, conscious and unhidden actions, behavior, and emotions.

Paradoxical Communication: Refers to the typical patterns of verbal and nonverbal communication between individuals and within families. It involves incongruent but consistent contradiction, qualification, or denial of previously made statements and actions and results in distrust, confusion, and ultimately meaningless communication.

Paranoid: Used as an adjective to describe unwarranted suspiciousness and distrust of others.

Personality: The characteristic way in which a person behaves; the deeply ingrained pattern of behavior that each person evolves, both consciously and unconsciously, as his style of life or way of being in adapting to his envoronment.*

Phenothiazines: The major group of psychotropic drugs used in the treatment of mental illness, chiefly the psychoses. Their chemical action is on the C.N.S.

Phobia: An irrational, persistent, obsessive intense fear of an object or situation, which results in increased anxiety and tension and which interferes with the individual's normal functioning.

Psychoanalysis: A form of psychotherapy developed by Freud, based on his theories of personality development and disorder, generally requiring basic commitments from the patient (analysand) to the therapist (analyst) regarding time, money, and procedure. The technique of psychoanalysis involves an examination of the free associations of a patient and the interpretation of his dreams, emotions, and behavior. Its focus is mainly on the way the ego handles the id tensions. Psychoanalysis is a lengthy, costly, esoteric treatment approach and is concerned only with the intrapsychic processes of the individual analysand. In psychoanalysis, success is measured by the degree of insight the patient is able to gain into the unconscious motivations of his behavior.

Psychodrama: A form of group psychotherapy developed by Moreno in which patients dramatize their emotional problems. By assuming roles in order to act out their conflicts they reveal repressed feelings which have been disturbing to them.

Psychogenic: Implies the causative factors of a symptom or illness are due to mental rather than organic factors.

Psychosis: A major mental illness characterized by any of the following symptoms: loss of contact with a denial of reality,
        bizarre thinking and behavior, delusions,
        hallucinations, regression, disorientation.
Intrapsychically, it results from the unconscious becoming conscious and taking over control of the individual. In psychosis the ego is overwhelmed by the id and the super-ego.

Psychotherapy: The treatment of mental disorders or a psychosomatic condition by psychologic methods using a variety of approaches, including: psychoanalysis, group therapy, family therapy, psychodrama, hypnotism, simple counseling, suggestion.

Reality: The way things actually are.

Reality Oriented Therapy: Refers to any therapeutic approach whose focus is on helping the patient to define his reality, to improve his ability to adjust and to function productively and satisfactorily within his real situation.

Schizophrenogenic: An adjective used to describe the object or situation which is felt to be causative in the development of schizophrenia.

Super-Ego: The third part of the Freudian personality theory, which guides and restrains, criticizes and punishes just as the parents did when the individual was a child. It is unconscious, and it is learned. Like the id, the super-ego also wants its own way. Is sometimes referred to as the conscience.

Symbiotic Tie: In family therapy this refers to a pathogenic relationship between the parent (usually the mother) and child which is characterized by retarded ego development and overdependence in the child.

Therapist: Refers to an individual who by reason of his/her training, experience and knowledge is able and willing to use his/her skills to assist patients in the recovery and maintenance of health.

Transactional Analysis: A psychodynamic approach that attempts to understand the interplay between individuals in terms of the roles they have been assigned, assumed, or play in their transactions with others.

Triad: In contrast to dyad, refers to relationship among three individuals.

Unconscious: The repository of those mental processes of which the individual is unaware. The repressed feelings, and their energy, are stored in the unconscious and directly influence the individual's behavior.

Word Salad: A jumbled mixture of words and phrases which have no meaning, and are illogical in their sequence. Seen most often in schizophrenia. (e.g., Backter dyce tonked up snorfel blend.)

Index